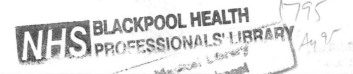

EXPLAINING CARDIAC SURGERY

Patient Assessment and Care

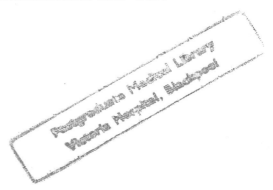

EXPLAINING CARDIAC SURGERY
Patient Assessment and Care

Russell Millner MD FRCS (CTh)
Consultant cardiothoracic surgeon
Victoria Hospital, Blackpool

Tom Treasure MS MD FRCS
Professor of cardiothoracic surgery
St George's Hospital, London

BMJ
Publishing
Group

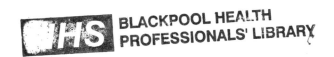
First published in 1995
by the BMJ Publishing Group, BMA House, Tavistock Square, London WC1H 9JR

British Library Cataloguing in Publication Data

A catalogue record for this book is available from the British Library

ISBN 0-7279-0853-7

Typeset by Apek Typesetters Ltd, Nailsea, Bristol
Printed and bound in Great Britain by Latimer Trend & Company Ltd., Plymouth

Contents

Preface   vii

1 Preoperative assessment of patients for cardiac surgery   1

2 Techniques in cardiac surgery   6

3 Myocardial protection   19

4 Early postoperative management   24

5 Surgery for coronary artery disease   44

6 Surgery for complications of ischaemic heart disease   66

7 Surgery for valvar heart disease   78

8 Surgical options in the management of heart and lung
   failure   105

9 Other cardiac lesions   130

10 Emergencies in cardiac surgery   139

11 Congenital heart disease   153

12 The postoperative period   170

Index   178

Preface

Since the development of modern techniques in cardiac surgery there has been a huge increase in the number of patients treated surgically for their heart disease. In the 1950s the operations were confined to treating congenital heart disease in children and simple procedures in adults, but during the last forty years many more adults have been treated. Initially operations were restricted to those with rheumatic heart disease, but during the last 20 years indications have been widened to include ischaemic heart disease, and more recently degenerative diseases of the cardiac valves. The surgical treatment of heart failure is also increasing, as reflected in the increasing demand for donor organs for both cardiac and pulmonary transplantation.

As an example, in the United Kingdom in 1990, 278 operations/million head of population were done for ischaemic heart disease in the NHS, compared with 107/million in 1982. This gives a total of 16 145 operations for ischaemic heart disease in 1990, of which 14 431 were isolated coronary artery bypasses, and the rest were combined procedures, generally with valve replacement. In comparison, in 1982 there was a total of 7403 operations for ischaemic heart disease and of these 6008 were isolated coronary artery bypasses. Parallel with this increase in work, there was increased pressure on beds and other facilities within the cardiothoracic units. This led to more rapid discharge of patients from these units, either transferred back to referring hospitals or discharged home or to convalescence. Consequently an increasing number of non-specialists are looking after these patients relatively early in their convalescence, at a time when there is still the potential for problems to occur.

In a wider sense though, there is a need for referring practitioners to understand clearly the procedures available. This is not just so that more patients who could benefit from operation are referred, but also so that both practitioners and their patients will better understand both the risks and the benefits not only of the operations themselves, but also of the separate procedures that make up the operation as a whole. For example, using the internal thoracic artery as a bypass graft has short term risks but long term benefits for most patients. They need to understand why the long term benefits outweigh the short term risks in general, and also be aware of the groups of patients in which this may not be so.

The main aim of this book is to provide a general overview of some of the techniques used in cardiac surgery. Secondly, we aim to set out the risk-benefit analysis of the commoner cardiac operations. Thirdly, we aim to answer the questions that patients repeatedly ask us during their postoperative visits — questions such as when can I drive, or fly, and what can I do to improve my chances of long term survival, and why is my leg numb?

We have not set out to produce a closely referenced text book for higher cardiac surgical trainees, but a guide for the wide range of medical, para-medical, and nursing staff who come into contact with these patients. Our aim is to demystify, illustrate, and explain what to us is a fascinating specialty.

RUSSELL MILLNER
TOM TREASURE

1 Preoperative assessment of patients for cardiac surgery

Essential investigations:

- Routine blood and urine tests
- Electrocardiogram (ECG)
- Chest x ray film
- Exercise ECG
- Echocardiogram (especially for valves or heart failure)
- Cardiac catheterisation

All patients referred for routine elective or urgent cardiac surgery will already have undergone extensive cardiological assessment, only the most dire emergency will be operated on without considerable preoperative investigation. The standard work-up includes taking of a history, physical examination and a number of investigations. Symptoms are commonly described in terms of the New York Heart Association Functional Classification (NYHA). An electrocardiogram (ECG), chest x ray film, full blood count, measurement of urea and electrolyte concentrations, liver function tests, clotting tests and hepatitis B antigen status are routine for all patients. Most will then go on to have one or more of the following more specialised investigations: exercise ECG, echocardiography, and cardiac catheterisation.

Electrocardiography

A baseline ECG is an essential part of a patient's management, because even if the tracing is within normal limits at rest, it provides a reference with which future examinations can be compared. An abnormal ECG can be

New York Heart Association Functional Classification:

Class 1

Patients with cardiac disease, but without resulting limitation of physical activity. Ordinary physical activity does not cause undue fatigue, palpitation, dyspnoea, or anginal pain.

Class 2

Patients with cardiac disease resulting in slight limitation of physical activity. They are comfortable at rest. Ordinary physical activity results in fatigue, palpitation, dyspnoea, or anginal pain.

Class 3

Patients with cardiac disease resulting in marked limitation of physical activity. They are comfortable at rest. Less than ordinary physical activity results in fatigue, palpitation, dyspnoea, or anginal pain.

Class 4

Patients with cardiac disease resulting in inability to carry on any physical activity without discomfort. Symptoms of cardiac insufficiency or of the anginal syndrome may be present even at rest. If any physical activity is undertaken discomfort is increased.

diagnostic on its own, or in conjunction with the elicited physical signs and chest x ray film. Often, though, in the investigation of patients presenting with angina it is the "stress ECG", usually recorded while the patient exercises on a treadmill at increasing rate and gradient, that provides the data to indicate that further investigation is warranted.

The commoner regimens are the Bruce protocol, and the modified Bruce protocol. In both protocols the patient exercises at different stages, each lasting three minutes. Assessment is based on the heart rate achieved by the patient, changes in the S-T segment on a continuous 12 lead ECG, and the onset of ectopic activity or arrhythmias. The patient's reason for stopping is recorded, and with modern equipment the protocol can be combined with a metabolic assessment of the patient's peak work load using the VO_2max. The exercise ECG does have risks, and should be done in an area where resuscitation equipment and trained personnel are immediately available.

Echocardiography

Echocardiography has become the mainstay of non-invasive investigation of valve disease of the heart and of disease of the great vessels. It is also of considerable importance in the assessment of cardiac function in patients with heart failure. In children with heart disease it may avoid the need for

Bruce protocol

Time (mins)	Stage	Speed (mph)	Slope (%)
0–3	1	1.7	10
3–6	2	2.6	12
6–9	3	3.4	14
9–12	4	4.2	16
12–15	5	5.0	18
15–18	6	5.5	20
18–21	7	6.0	21

cardiac catheterisation, and for others it is used as an adjunct to invasive procedures. There are two types of echocardiography, M mode and cross-sectional, and the role of colour flow Doppler processing is increasing in importance. Echocardiography can be undertaken by either the transthoracic or transoesophageal routes in most patients, and its use during the operation with a sterile epicardial transducer is increasing.

Transoesophageal echocardiography

Transoesophageal echocardiography is extremely useful in the assessment of mitral and aortic valve disease, as well as disease of both the ascending and descending aorta. It is less useful in the region of the aortic arch because the air filled trachea is between the aortic arch and the oesophagus. Echocardiography is particularly useful for emergencies, and for non-invasive assessment of the aorta in cases of suspected aortic dissection. It also helps to distinguish between postinfarction ventricular septal rupture, postinfarction papillary muscle rupture, and mitral regurgitation.

Modified Bruce protocol

Time (mins)	Stage	Speed (mph)	Slope (%)
0–3	1	1.7	0
3–6	2	1.7	5
6–9	3	1.7	10
9–12	4	2.5	12
12–15	5	3.4	14
15–18	6	4.2	16
18–21	7	5.0	18

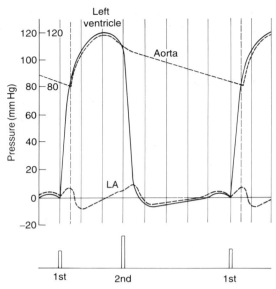

Figure 1.1 Normal pressures within the left ventricle and left atrium (timed against first and second heart sounds).

Cardiac catheterisation

Cardiac catheterisation is the mainstay of diagnosis in cardiac disease, and numerous techniques are being developed in which it is part of a therapeutic procedure. Almost all patients will have had a cardiac catheter before their referral for operation, the only exceptions are some infants and neonates with congenital heart disease and some young patients with isolated valve disease confirmed on good quality echocardiographic examination.

The essentials of the technique are the introduction of a catheter into the heart, the recording of pressures within the heart and great vessels, and the injection of contrast into the appropriate cavities and vessels under radiographic control and recording. This provides haemodynamic data, particularly aortic and left ventricular pressures, which will (if relevant) be augmented with data from catheterisation of the right heart. These data are used to assess left ventricular function before operation (see fig 1.1).

Left ventricular angiograms

The left ventricular angiogram gives further data about overall and segmental left ventricular function, together with an assessment of mitral regurgitation if present. The images are an essential part of the investigation of patients with suspected ischaemic heart disease. Much of the decision making hangs on the state of the left ventricle and the anatomy of the coronary arteries at angiography.

Isotope and other studies

Where the decision to operate or maintain medical treatment is still not clear and review of the patient's symptoms is unhelpful, then various isotope studies are used. In particular, thallium scans are used to look for evidence of areas of reversible myocardial ischaemia, and multiple gated acquisition (MUGA) scans as an alternative assessment of left ventricular ejection fraction. Ultrafast ECG gated computerised tomography (CT) and ECG gated nuclear magnetic resonance imaging (MRI), both with the use of the appropriate contrast media, are being increasingly used. Certainly in diseases of the aorta both CT and MRI produce clear images, with diagnostic yields that are comparable with those supplied by conventional cardiac catheterisation. MRI has been used in the assessment of bypass graft patency after operation.

Conclusion

For the foreseeable future, cardiac catheterisation will be the mainstay of invasive cardiology. The general techniques of cardiac catheterisation are being expanded as cardiology becomes more invasive, and the technology becomes more refined. Balloon coronary angioplasty is an established treatment that is being augmented by techniques such as laser angioplasty, rotablation, and coronary stenting. Other allied techniques include percutaneous balloon dilatation of the pulmonary valve, together with aortic coarctation in children and percutaneous balloon dilatation of the mitral valve in adults. Techniques for the percutaneous closure of atrial and ventricular septal defects are also being developed.

There are a number of other techniques currently being used for research that will probably find their way into clinical practice during the next few years; these include angioscopy and endovascular ultrasonography. Angioscopy, as its name suggests, is the insertion of a fibre-optic scope into the lumen of an artery. Its main limitation is the difficulty of providing a bloodless viewing field. Endovascular ultrasonography is the insertion of an ultrasound transducer mounted on a catheter into the lumen of a blood vessel. The potential roles of both this and angioscopy seem at present to lie more in the realms of invasive cardiology and angioplasty than cardiac surgery itself.

2 Techniques in cardiac surgery

- Surgical access to the heart
- Cardiopulmonary bypass
- Total circulatory arrest
- External anatomy of an adult heart

Surgical access to the heart

Over the years a number of different incisions have been used to gain access to the heart and great vessels, but a median sternotomy is now the most favoured route of access to the heart for most operations. There are occasional exceptions in paediatric surgery and reoperations. These are either for cosmetic reasons (for example, in young girls), or to attempt to lessen the impact of adhesions from a previous operation. For a median sternotomy the patient is intubated, and the appropriate monitoring lines inserted. The patient is placed supine on the operating field, the skin is prepared with antiseptic solution, and the operative field draped. The skin is incised in the midline from the manubrium to the xiphisternum, and the incision deepened through the subcutaneous tissue to the bone. Generally there is no muscle in the midline, though occasionally the origins of pectoralis major are asymmetrical. The sternum is divided in the midline with a saw. Haemostasis of the sternal edges is secured, and the sternal edges separated with a spreader. This exposes the pleurae which are in turn swept aside to expose the pericardium. The thymus is usually mobilised to expose the innominate vein, and with this in view the pericardium is opened to expose the heart (see fig 2.1).

(a)

(b)

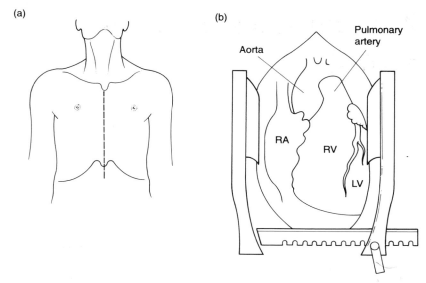

Figure 2.1 The standard incision for cardiac surgery is the median sternotomy. The sternum is cut exactly in the midline with a saw (a) and the two edges are held apart by a powerful geared retractor to expose the heart (b). All the vessels and chambers can be reached by this approach.

At the end of the operation drains are placed into the pleural, pericardial, and mediastinal spaces, as appropriate. The pericardium is usually left open, although it may be closed in some cases. Haemostasis is secured and the sternum closed with about six number 5 stainless steel wire loops. The subcutaneous layers are usually closed with an absorbable suture, and the skin closed with an absorbable subcuticular suture. Pacing wires may also be placed on the epicardial surface of the heart, either for use in weaning the patient from bypass or as an insurance policy for the management of bradycardias in the early postoperative period. The drains are usually removed within 24-36 hours, and the pacing wires after about five days.

Cardiopulmonary bypass

What it is

Cardiopulmonary bypass is the means by which a patient's circulation is supported during operations on the heart and great vessels. It is not unusual though for the term "bypass" in cardiology and cardiac surgery to be misunderstood for "coronary artery bypass" so for clarity the full term "cardiopulmonary bypass" will be used in this section.

7

Cardiopulmonary bypass

- Blood from atrium into reservoir
- Oxygenation of blood
- Heat exchanger
- Blood pumped back into aorta
- Blood scavenged by suckers and vents

Cardiopulmonary bypass was developed experimentally during and after the second world war, though the first operation done under cardiopulmonary bypass did not take place until 1953 when Gibbon repaired an atrial septal defect. Since then there have been considerable improvements in the materials and technology involved in cardiopulmonary bypass so that today it is unusual to have a mishap that is related to the cardiopulmonary bypass equipment itself.

How it works

The cardiopulmonary bypass pump is usually used to take over both the pumping action of the heart and the gas-exchange features of the lungs. By regulating the total gas and by varying the proportions of air and oxygen in the mixture it is possible to manipulate the values of PaO_2 and $PaCO_2$ in the blood stream. It is also possible to add anaesthetic vaporisers to the circuit to aid in the maintenance of anaesthesia while the patient is on cardiopulmonary bypass. A typical cardiopulmonary bypass circuit is illustrated in figure 2.2. The circuit will have a number of separate components, including cannulas and their connecting tubing, a reservoir, a number of pumps, and an oxygenator.

Anticoagulation

As blood must be removed from the vascular system into prosthetic material such as the cannulas, bypass tubing, reservoirs and oxygenators, it must be anti-coagulated. Failure to do this results in catastrophic clotting within the bypass circuits, with the further possibility of embolisation of debris into the arterial system. Heparin in a dose of 3 mg/kg is given at least two minutes either before cannulation, or before blood is sucked back into the reservoir of the cardiopulmonary bypass machine. Generally the activated clotting time (ACT) is measured before cannulation and should be at least 400 seconds at that point. Further increments of heparin are given during the bypass run if the ACT falls below this level. At the end of bypass and after the venous cannula has been removed, the heparin is reversed by protamine

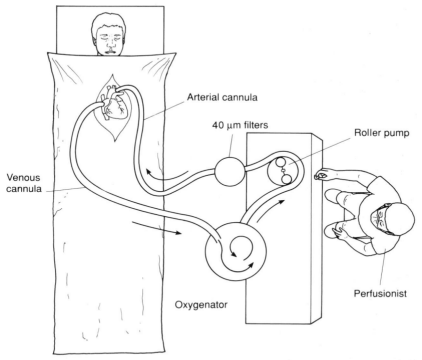

Figure 2.2 The essential components of the bypass circuit. A pipe about 1.5 cm in diameter drains all the patient's blood from the venous circuit to a reservoir from where it runs through an oxygenator. It is pressurised by the roller pump and driven through a filter before being returned to the arterial circulation through a pipe about 1 cm in diameter.

sulphate, mg for mg, after which the ACT is checked again and further protamine sulphate is given if necessary.

Cannulation

In a typical circuit blood is drained by gravity from the right atrium into a reservoir. According to the operative requirements, blood is either drained from the right atrium into the cardiopulmonary bypass circuit through a single cannula, or each vena cava is cannulated separately. A single cannula is used for most closed cardiac operations, such as coronary artery bypass and for operations on the aortic valve and ascending aorta. This cannula is generally inserted through a purse string suture in the right atrial appendage.

9

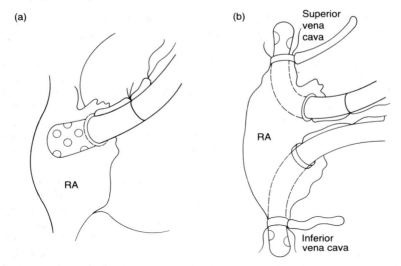

Figure 2.3 The venous blood can be drained from the patient with a single large pipe in the right atrium (a). For more complex operations, or when the right atrium itself must be entered, the pipes are positioned separately in the inferior vena cava and superior vena cava (b).

If it is necessary to open either the left atrium or the left ventricle it is usual to place two separate cannulas, one in the superior vena cava and one in the inferior vena cava. The cannula in the superior vena cava is also inserted through a purse string suture placed in the right atrial appendage and then guided into the superior vena cava. The cannula in the inferior vena cava is inserted through a purse string suture placed low down in the right atrial free wall, generally a centimetre or so above the insertion of the inferior vena cava into the right atrium. If it is necessary to open the right atrium itself, tapes are passed around the superior and inferior vena cavas and passed through plastic "snuggers" so that the vessel wall can be gathered around the cannulas, ensuring that all the blood flows into the cannulas and preventing air passing back from the open right atrium into the cardiopulmonary bypass circuit (see fig 2.3).

The blood draining from the right atrium passes through the cannulas and the connecting tubing and then into a reservoir which allows blood to be stored within the bypass circuit. This is important as the vascular tone of the patient will vary during the bypass run, and at different times different volumes of blood will be required to maintain appropriate pressures within the venous and arterial systems of the patient and flows from the bypass circuit. The reservoir is also a convenient point at which further amounts of fluid may be added to the bypass circuit if required, together with any drugs.

From this reservoir blood passes both through an oxygenator where gas exchange occurs and through a pump before it passes back into the patient's arterial circulation (see fig 2.2).

The arterial return from the bypass pump is usually through a cannula placed, through a purse string suture, into the distal part of the ascending aorta or the proximal part of the aortic arch (fig 2.4). This allows the whole of the cardiopulmonary bypass cannulation to be done through a median sternotomy without any other incisions. It is quite possible in an emergency, such as for a dissection of the ascending aorta or if a major structure has been damaged during a repeat sternotomy, to institute cardiopulmonary bypass rapidly through cannulation of the common femoral artery.

There are occasional circumstances when the common femoral artery is cannulated electively, and indeed if the common femoral vein is also cannulated it is possible to achieve cardiopulmonary bypass before opening the chest. This is occasionally done in reoperations when particular difficulty is anticipated in reopening the old sternotomy incision. Patients with appreciably raised right atrial pressure, and those with a dilated ascending aorta or a mycotic aneurysm are at increased risk of damage during sternal

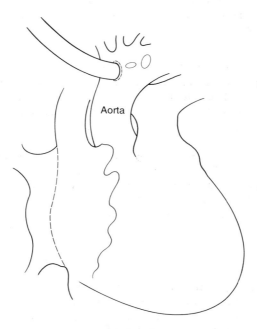

Aorta

Figure 2.4 Arterial cannulation. Arterial blood is returned to the patient through a single pipe that is inserted into the ascending aorta. Occasionally arterial return is into the femoral artery rather than the ascending aorta.

11

reentry, and femoral artery cannulation is commonly used. Femoral artery cannulation is also done routinely for patients with aortic dissections.

Oxygenators

The function of the oxygenator is, as its name suggests, to transfer oxygen into the blood stream. It also removes carbon dioxide from the blood stream thereby taking over the gas exchange functions of the lungs.

There are two general types of oxygenator in current use, one known as a "bubble oxygenator" and the second as a "membrane oxygenator". The bubble oxygenators are older and their use is gradually declining; they work by bubbling a mixture of oxygen and air through the blood stream, usually as it passes through the reservoir. As this creates a considerable amount of foaming, measures have to be taken in the design of the oxygenator to prevent gaseous microembolisation when using this technique and it is usual also to have an additional filter on the arterial return line of the bypass circuit to further reduce gaseous microembolisation.

Membrane oxygenators do not have a direct interface between the gas mixture and the blood stream; instead, gas transfer occurs across a gas permeable membrane separating the gas flow from the blood stream. There are two main types of membrane oxygenator in current use — in one the blood gas interface occurs across sheets, with the gas on one side and the blood on the other side of the membrane, and in the second the blood gas interface occurs through hollow fibres, with the gas passing through the interior of the fibre and the blood passing around the fibre. In some oxygenators the blood passed through the interior of the fibre and the gas passed around the fibre, but these have now been discontinued for technical reasons.

Bypass pumps

The arterial pump will be placed either just before or just after the oxygenator in the circuit, depending on the type of oxygenator used. The pump will usually be placed before a membrane oxygenator but after a bubble oxygenator, because there is an increased resistance to blood flow through the membrane oxygenator. There are two major types of arterial pumps in current use. The first are the roller pumps, in which a rotating head squeezes blood through silastic tubing in a sweeping action. In the second, the constrained vortex pumps, blood is accelerated by a spinning turbine, the theoretical advantage being that less damage is done to the blood as it passes through the pump. The advantages of the roller pumps are that they are cheaper because they require fewer disposable materials, and they can be made to generate a pulsatile blood flow.

The blood is again filtered between the oxygenator and the arterial circulation to reduce the possibility of transfusing particulate debris and gaseous microemboli back into the patient.

Vents and suckers

To minimise the amount of blood and other fluids that have to be added to the patient either during or after cardiopulmonary bypass, blood that is collecting around the heart in the pericardial or pleural cavities is sucked up and returned to the reservoir by a separate pump and tubing system known simply as suckers. Other pipes – vents – also drain blood back into the reservoir. The vents drain blood from within the cavities of the heart but are otherwise exactly the same as the suckers.

Common sites through which to place vents include the apex of the left ventricle, the right superior pulmonary vein and across the mitral valve into the cavity of the left ventricle, the aortic root proximal to the cross-clamp and from the pulmonary trunk. The general function of a vent is to stop the heart filling with blood and becoming distended. Aortic root vents are also used in coronary artery surgery to help keep the anastomosis clear of blood during the construction of the coronary grafts (see fig 2.5).

Who runs it?

The cardiopulmonary bypass equipment is set up and run by technicians who are known colloquially as perfusionists. They undergo a training course to Higher National Certificate in medical physics and physiological measurement and are licensed in the United Kingdom by the Society of Perfusionists as Accredited Clinical Perfusionists. They are primarily responsible for setting up and running the bypass equipment, but during the operation they will liaise closely with both the anaesthetist and surgeons on the management of blood pressure, pump flows, and the use of both vasodilating and vasoconstricting agents.

The risks of cardiopulmonary bypass

It is inevitable that when a patient is connected to a machine there are risks. When both the circulation and ventilation are interrupted and the patient is completely dependent on the machine the potential for disaster is further increased. Fortunately disasters caused by or associated with cardiopulmonary bypass are rare, and can be divided into those caused by the equipment itself, and those during cannulation of the patient for bypass.

In the latter group, the most common are bleeding from cannulation sites and arrhythmias as a result of handling the heart during cannulation. In practical terms arrhythmias are common during atrial cannulation and usually unimportant, while serious bleeding from cannulation sites is

13

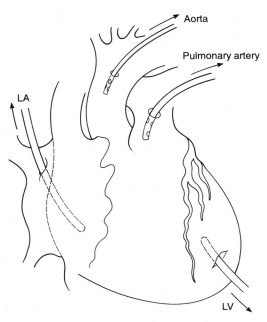

Figure 2.5 "Venting" the heart during cardiopulmonary bypass. The fibrillating or asystolic heart is at risk of dilating, which stretches the muscles and creates tension in the subendocardium and ischaemia. This is avoided as necessary by venting with tubes inserted in one of the sites that will decompress the left side.

uncommon but has the potential to cause serious trouble. The other serious complication arises when there is difficulty in cannulating the ascending aorta because of atheroma in it. Disturbing a plaque during aortic cannulation may cause a stroke. This devastating complication should be avoided by meticulous attention to palpating the chosen site of cannulation before the purse string suture is inserted.

The common complications related to the bypass circuit itself are those of platelet depletion, red cell damage, and complement activation. They are all measurable, and are not usually clinically relevant. In the occasional patient a particularly profound depletion of platelets, together with an impairment of platelet function may be associated with severe postoperative haemorrhage. The most devastating complication of cardiopulmonary bypass is, however, the introduction of air into the arterial circulation. Fortunately in modern practice this is exceedingly rare because of the increasing use of membrane oxygenators, the vigilance of the perfusionists, and the use of low level alarms and constrained vortex pumps. What is more common is the production of microemboli of air during cannulation of the arterial circulation; although

14

this is rarely clinically evident, it is associated with some of the short term and reversible neuropsychological effects of bypass, such as poor memory and concentration, which are seen in a number of patients after cardiac surgery.

Total circulatory arrest

For complex operations, particularly in infants and neonates but also for those on the ascending aorta and aortic arch in adults, the body temperature may be reduced to about 12–15°C. At this temperature the entire circulation can be interrupted completely for periods of up to 45 minutes. It has also been suggested that by lowering the basal metabolic rate (BMR) by cooling, the flow rate of the cardiopulmonary bypass circuit can be reduced with possible benefits including a reduced embolic load to the brain. This allows complex procedures to be undertaken which would otherwise be technically extremely difficult, if not impossible. It is reasonably safe, particularly for less than 30 minutes of circulatory arrest, but the evidence both from studies of outcome and neuropsychometric studies shows that the longer the period of hypothermic arrest the higher the risk of the patient sustaining cerebral damage. Clearly this is a classic example of the expected benefits of the surgical repair having to be balanced against the risks of the operative technique.

A number of methods have been developed to try and reduce the incidence of cerebral damage during circulatory arrest. Infants, and in some units adults, have ice or cooling blankets around their heads. Pharmacological methods include high doses of thiopentone, (up to 2 g intravenously just before circulatory arrest). Mannitol and steroids and nimodipine are also given sometimes. Surgical methods include continuous antegrade cerebral perfusion by separate cannulation of the innominate and left common carotid arteries, or continuous retrograde cerebral perfusion through the superior vena cava. Currently the numbers of patients operated on with any particular technique are too small for one to have achieved particular prominence, except the use of large doses of thiopentone.

Total circulatory arrest is usually combined with cardioplegic arrest of the heart.

External anatomy of an adult heart

The heart is a hollow muscular organ sited in the chest in the middle mediastinum entirely contained by the pericardial cavity, and bordering on the lungs laterally, the diaphragm inferiorly, and the spinal column, oesophagus, tracheal carina, and descending aorta posteriorly. The sternum is anterior and the costal cartilages and medial ends of the 4th to 7th ribs on the left. The great vessels and thymus lie superiorly.

The average normal adult heart measures about 12 cm from base to apex, 6 cm in the anteroposterior direction, and 9 cm transversely at its widest point. An average normal female heart will weigh about 230–280 g and an average normal male heart about 280–340 g. The walls of the normal right and left atria are both little more than 1 mm thick, whilst the normal right ventricle is about 3 mm thick and the normal left ventricle about 9 to 12 mm.

At sternotomy, little can usually be seen of the left ventricle or left atrium, and most of the ventricular muscle seen is right ventricle. On the right side the superior vena cava emerges from the pericardial reflection and descends for an inch or so to the right atrium. On the anterior surface at the junction of the superior vena cava and the trabeculated portion of the right atrial appendage is a slightly yellow crescent of tissue, about 3 × 8 mm and often marked by a small artery; this is the sinus node. Behind the junction of the superior vena cava and the right atrium is the right pulmonary artery and at operation this can be displayed by retracting the aorta to the left and the superior vena cava to the right. Below the right atrium, the inferior vena cava emerges through the diaphragm and joins the right atrium. A groove that runs from behind the superior vena cava to behind the junction of the inferior vena cava and the right atrium shows the surface marking of the interatrial septum. If the right atrium is displaced to the left, the left atrium can be seen behind it, together with the junction of the right superior and right inferior pulmonary veins and the left atrium. The junction of the free wall of the right atrium and the right ventricle marks the right atrioventricular groove, and the main right coronary artery runs here. The coronary sinus lies below and behind the left of the junction of the inferior vena cava and the right atrium. If the acute margin of the heart is retracted forward, the posterior descending artery in the posterior interventricular groove can be identified. If the heart is retracted to the right the left anterior descending artery can be seen in the anterior interventricular groove, together with the tip of the left atrial appendage to the left side of the pulmonary trunk.

If the right atrium is opened, the atrial septum and orifices of the superior and inferior vena cavas can be seen. The tricuspid valve marks the junction with the cavity of the right ventricle. The triangle formed between the septal leaflet of the tricuspid valve, the mouth of the coronary sinus, and a ridge of connective tissue running from the coronary sinus (the tendon of Todaro) is an important anatomical landmark. At the apex of the triangle lies the atrioventricular node from which the bundle of His arises before it runs into the membranous septum. The atrial septum has a convex groove, which is the limbus of the fossa ovalis and marks the limit of the embryological septum secundum. It is the site of a classic secundum atrial septal defect.

The right ventricle is marked on the surface by the sinuses of the pulmonary valve above, the right atrioventricular groove on the right, the posterior descending coronary artery below, and to the left by the left anterior descending coronary artery. When seen through the tricuspid valve, or if opened, it is partly separated into an inlet part and an outlet part. This separation is marked by a muscular ridge, the supraventricular crest; the inlet part has rough walls, and the outlet part the infundibulum, has smooth walls. This leads up to the pulmonary valve. There are two valves associated with the right ventricle, the inlet atrioventricular (or tricuspid) valve, and the outlet pulmonary valve. These are described in more detail in chapter 7.

The pulmonary trunk runs upwards and backwards, rotating to the left of the ascending aorta before bifurcating into the right pulmonary and left pulmonary arteries. The right pulmonary artery runs behind the ascending aorta and inferior vena cava and in front of the right main bronchus into the right chest, and the left pulmonary artery passes in front of the descending aorta and right main bronchus into the left chest.

The left atrium lies immediately in front of the oesophagus, and receives the pulmonary veins. At operation, if the right atrium is retracted to the left, the superior and inferior pulmonary veins can be identified, together with the interatrial septum. An incision can be made here to approach the mitral valve. The roof of the left atrium can be seen by retracting the superior vena cava to the right and the ascending aorta to the left, and if the heart is retracted to the right, the left atrial appendage can be seen along the right side of the pulmonary trunk.

The left ventricle is more conical than the right, and the walls are considerably thicker. On transverse section it is circular, and the right ventricle is seen as a crescent attached to the septal side of the circle. The interventricular septum is a thick muscular structure, except in its upper part, (just below the junction of the right coronary and non-coronary cusps of the aortic valve) where there is a fibrous area called the membranous septum. This area is of surgical importance as the bundle of His runs through here and damage (for instance, during aortic valve replacement) will cause complete heart block.

The interior of the left ventricle is marked by a number of structures. The left atrioventricular or mitral orifice lies below and slightly to the left of the aortic orifice, and is oval in shape, while the aortic orifice is circular. These valves are described in more detail in chapter 7.

The ascending aorta arises from the left ventricle immediately distal to the cusps of the aortic valve. It passes obliquely upwards, in front and to the right before continuing as the aortic arch, which curves around the left pulmonary artery and left main bronchus to continue as the descending aorta. It has five branches during this course; the left and right coronary arteries, the right brachiocephalic trunk, the left common carotid artery, and the left subclavian artery.

The coronary arteries are the first branches of the aorta. The left main coronary artery arises in the left sinus of Valsava (a dilatation in the root of the ascending aorta) and passes between the pulmonary artery and the left atrial appendage to reach the left atrioventricular groove. Its usual length is 1 to 2 cm before it divides into the left anterior descending and left circumflex arteries. The right coronary artery arises in the right sinus of Valsava before running into the right atrioventricular groove. The coronary arteries are described in more detail in chapter 5.

The anatomy of the conducting system is of considerable importance in cardiac surgery. The sinus node lies on the anterior surface of the right atrium at the junction of the superior vena cava and the trabeculated portion of the right atrial appendage. The atrioventricular node lies on the right atrial side of the central fibrous body at the apex of the triangle formed between the septal leaflet of the tricuspid valve, the mouth of the coronary sinus, and a ridge of fibrous tissue running from the coronary sinus (the tendon of Todaro).

The bundle of His is a direct continuation of the atrioventricular node and passes through the right trigone of the central fibrous body to the postero-inferior margin of the membranous septum. It then passes along the crest of the muscular septum, and below the commissure between the right and non-coronary cusps it gives off the left bundle branch after which the remaining fibres make up the right bundle branch. The left bundle branch fans out over the left ventricular septal surface, usually with anterior and posterior subdivisions. The anterior hemifascicle runs towards the base of the anterolateral papillary muscle, while the posterior hemifascicle runs towards the base of the posteromedial papillary muscle. The right bundle arises from the bundle of His in the region of the anteroinferior margin of the membranous septum and passes along the right ventricular side of the interventricular septum, below the medial papillary muscle to the base of the anterior papillary muscle, where its fibres then fan out to supply the muscle of the right ventricle.

3 Myocardial protection

It is often necessary to stop the heart beating, sometimes for a long period, to provide a still field in which to operate. It may also be necessary to stop blood flowing through the coronary arteries, particularly in coronary artery surgery when the anastomosis may be to a vessel of little over 1 mm in diameter. For operations in which the heart must be opened it is often a requirement to cross–clamp the ascending aorta either to prevent air entering the arterial system, or simply to allow the operation to be done. During transplantation the heart may be completely without a blood supply for many hours while it is in transit. In all these cases technical strategies must be employed to minimise the damage to the heart during the periods when its blood supply is interrupted.

There are a number of ways in which the heart can be operated on in a still and relatively bloodless field. The most common include cold cardioplegic arrest, intermittent ischaemic arrest (syn cross–clamp fibrillation), and continuous perfusion of the heart. Each of these techniques has its own variants, its attractions, and its limitations. There are differences among the techniques, and there is controversy about which is superior. In the meantime development of old and the introduction of new methods of myocardial protection continues.

Cardioplegia

To work successfully and accurately on the heart it is usually necessary to isolate it from its blood supply for a time. Cardioplegia is the technique of using either a crystalloid solution, or more recently blood, to deliver a high concentration of potassium to the heart. This arrests the heart in diastole, leaving it flaccid and still, which is excellent for meticulous operating. The solution is usually cooled to about 4°C to slow myocardial metabolism while the heart is isolated from its blood supply.

With appropriate precautions the heart can be made ischaemic for a considerable time, and still function adequately when it is eventually reperfused. In routine clinical practice it can be ischaemic for up to two hours or so, while for transplantation times above four hours are not unusual. The difference is that while the heart is in the body it is warmed and receives a collateral flow from the rest of the body. While it is being transported for transplantation however, it is kept in a container of ice at around 0°C for four hours or longer.

Types of cardioplegic arrest

Though there is increasing interest and experience in using blood as the delivery system for the cardioplegia, most clinical experience has been with crystalloid solutions (usually compound sodium lactate). Until recently the most common method was cold crystalloid cardioplegic arrest. A bolus of potassium–rich crystalloid perfusate, usually one litre for an adult, is used to produce diastolic arrest of the heart while the low temperature of the perfusate is used to preserve the heart by cooling and minimise the damage produced by a prolonged period of ischaemia. When blood rather than crystalloid is used as the delivery medium this technique is known as cold blood cardioplegic arrest. The bolus infusion is repeated at intervals, usually of about 30 minutes or earlier if electrical activity is seen on the ECG. The supplement is usually 300 to 500 ml of the same solution. In its simplest form the perfusate, known as cardioplegia, is injected into the ascending aorta under pressure after the aorta has been cross–clamped more distally. This cross–clamp isolates the heart from the arterial circulation, and renders it completely ischaemic.

By perfusing the ascending aorta with cardioplegia, below the cross–clamp and if the aortic valve is functioning, the cardioplegia is forced directly into the coronary arteries and rapidly delivered to the heart (fig 3.1).

This is known as antegrade cold cardioplegia, the usual temperature of the cardioplegia at the time of delivery being about 0–4°C, and the target being to reduce the temperature of the myocardium to about 10–15°C. For convenience the temperature of the interventricular septum is measured and considered to represent the myocardium as a whole. The cooling effect of the

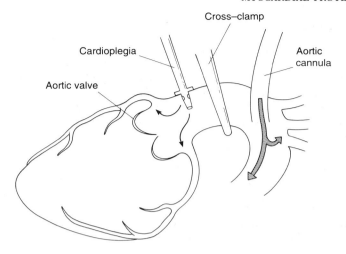

Figure 3.1 Arresting the heart with cardioplegic solution. The body is perfused with blood from the bypass machine (large hatched arrow). There is a cross–clamp on the aorta and proximal to that a small cannula is placed to perfuse the coronary arteries separately. Blood with a higher than normal concentration of potassium is infused to arrest the heart and the temperature can be lowered substantially to aid protection.

cardioplegic solution can be augmented by filling the pericardial cavity with either slush or ice-cold crystalloid solution. Slush takes up proportionately far more energy than the solution, and is far more effective in cooling the myocardium, so it is preferred by many surgeons. Because of concerns about uneven distribution of cardioplegia to the heart, particularly in patients with obstructive coronary artery disease, there has been considerable interest in augmenting this technique with cold cardioplegia infused retrogradely into the coronary sinus. This technique, known as retrograde cold cardioplegia, is often used in conjunction with antegrade cold cardioplegia. There is some evidence that oxygenating and filtering a crystalloid cardioplegic solution increases its efficacy and safety.

Cardioplegia solutions

A standard solution for cardioplegia is given in the box, though this is only one of a number that are used worldwide. Blood cardioplegia is similar, except that the crystalloid solution is replaced by blood. At its simplest, Hartmann's solution is replaced by the patient's own blood drawn into a separate reservoir from the heart-lung bypass machine rapidly at the onset of bypass, and cooled down to 4°C. A concentrated solution of the agents used to make up crystalloid cardioplegia is added. The solution thus produced,

21

St Thomas's Cardioplegia

	mmol/l
Sodium chloride	144.3
Potassium chloride	19.6
Magnesium chloride	15.7
Calcium chloride	2.2
Procaine hydrochloride	0.05

blood cardioplegia, is infused in exactly the same way as crystalloid cardioplegia, producing what are known as antegrade cold blood cardioplegia and retrograde cold blood cardioplegia; like crystalloid cardioplegia they are often used together.

Cooling the patient

At the same time as the heart is cooled locally, the patient is also cooled by lowering the temperature of the blood that flows from the heart-lung bypass pump. For cold cardioplegic arrest most surgeons reduce the patient's temperature to between 26° and 28°C. The rationale for this is not only to reduce the amount of heat delivered to the heart from non-coronary collateral blood flow, but also to reduce the amount of heat delivered to the heart from the descending thoracic aorta which lies immediately behind the heart and which receives the arterial blood return from the cardiopulmonary bypass circuit. It has also been suggested that by lowering the basal metabolic rate through cooling, the flow rate of the cardiopulmonary bypass circuit can be reduced, with possible benefits including a reduced embolic load on the brain.

Warm blood reperfusion

Blood cardioplegia is further modified by techniques to increase its effectiveness; one of these is warm blood reperfusion. After the completion of the operation and before the cross–clamp is released, the heart is given a further infusion of blood cardioplegia, but this time at normal body temperature of 37°C, and with the addition of the amino acids L-glutamate and aspartate. The purpose is for the heart to reconstruct its energy stores while it is still asystolic and before it has to start work.

A version of this technique currently being explored is the continuous delivery of warm blood cardioplegia to the aortic root while the heart is maintained in asystolic arrest and the patient is maintained at normal body temperature. Though this looks at first sight to be a good alternative, there are a number of theoretical and practical problems.

Continuous coronary perfusion

For many years, a number of surgeons have used continuous perfusion of blood directly into the coronary orifices during aortic valve operations, and continuous perfusion of blood directly into the aortic root below the cross–clamp during mitral valve operations. This has allowed the heart to beat while it is opened, and the flow of blood can be temporarily interrupted for difficult parts of the procedure. The ischaemia that results from interrupting the coronary perfusion is minimised by doing the operation under moderate hypothermia, with the patient cooled down to about 31°C.

Intermittent ischaemic arrest

Another technique that is used for coronary artery surgery is intermittent ischaemic arrest, also known as cross–clamp fibrillation. The patient is cooled to about 31–32°C, the heart is then arrested by inducing ventricular fibrillation electrically, and the aorta is cross–clamped, making the heart ischaemic. Because the duration of ischaemia is limited to about 10 minutes each time, and the heart is reperfused between episodes of ischaemia, this technique is highly effective for coronary artery surgery. Interestingly, there is now some evidence that the heart may be preconditioned to any particular episode of ischaemia by a previous episode of ischaemia. This technique tends to be used by more experienced surgeons, however, although there is currently somewhat of a resurgence of interest in it.

4 Early postoperative management

- Intensive care unit
  Monitoring
- Common problems
  Special measures
  Airway management
  Treatment of respiratory dysfunction
  Arrhythmias
- Renal support
- Other complications
- The future

Intensive care unit (and high dependency unit)

The intensive care unit can be stressful for both patients and relatives. In many units patients who are to undergo elective operations will have been shown round the intensive care unit, usually the night before the operation. For some this helps to allay their anxiety, but there are others who still awake profoundly agitated. Most intensive care units operate an open visiting policy, though limited to two close relatives at a time, and this together with the fact that the stay is usually short helps to lessen apprehension in both the patient and the relatives. It is often better to advise relatives to telephone rather than visit, as this produces less disturbance in the unit and reduces the exposure of the relatives to a potentially stressful environment. It is usually worth pointing out that many patients have little recall of their night in the intensive care unit, and are usually moved out rapidly the next morning.

In the early hours after operation many, though by no means all, patients undergo a period of elective ventilation, during which time their general cardiovascular state is assessed and in particular the possibility of excessive bleeding is eliminated. After this patients are allowed to wake up gradually and breathe for themselves. During this time they will have cardiovascular variables, together with airway pressures and blood gases monitored, usually with continuous arterial oxygen saturation through a pulse oximeter. As the patients wake up, they gradually start to take breaths for themselves. When they are able to maintain their own airways satisfactorily with adequate respiratory function then they will be weaned from the ventilator and extubated.

Monitoring

The intensive care unit has two main functions; simple postoperative recovery for most patients, and true intensive care for comparatively few. Particularly the relatively fit patients having coronary artery surgery should realise that the intensive care unit is misnamed. These patients need intensive monitoring, and their usual requirements are analgesia, vasodilators, appropriate volume replacement, and diuretics, generally in that order. These requirements can usually be fulfilled in a ward that would be better named a high dependency unit, and in most units there is a tendency for an increasing amount of the work load to go straight from the operating theatre to the high dependency unit. Sometimes this will follow a stay of two or three hours in the theatre recovery room, and sometimes after a short stay in the intensive care unit before extubation.

There are a number of physiological measurements that must be made in a patient who has just had a cardiac operation, and they fall into groups such as haemodynamic, respiratory, renal and so on. There is a considerable degree of overlap between groups—for example, urine output is relevant to both the renal and haemodynamic groups. From these measurements, trends in a patient's performance over time can be identified.

The monitoring of trends is the main function of the intensive care unit for most patients. In simple terms, if the trends are moving in the right direction then a "hands off" approach is suitable; if not, a focused approach to the patient's problems is necessary.

One tends to discuss trends in various individual systems (such as cardiovascular or renal), but clearly the overall view requires integration of all the data before changes in management are considered. For example, it is as inappropriate to give loop diuretics for a low urine output when the patient is hypovolaemic, as it is to give a further volume load to a hypertensive patient with adequate central venous pressure and a low urine output.

25

Cardiac variables monitored

- Heart rate
- Heart rhythm
- Blood pressure
  Systemic arterial
  Pulmonary arterial and wedge
  Central venous
- Rate of bleeding from chest drains

Heart rate, blood pressure, central venous pressure

The measurement of heart rate, arterial blood pressure, and central venous pressure is the core of monitoring. The heart rate is dependent on several factors, including preoperative β blockade, transient or permanent operative damage, and postoperative events such as hypovolaemia and agitation. A trend towards increasing heart rate suggests relative hypovolaemia, myocardial damage, or awareness. A fall in heart rate from an increased reading to a more normal range after the appropriate treatment would be usual.

Monitoring arterial blood pressure is important because it provides not only an instantaneous measure of cardiac performance but also, through the recording of trends, an index of change in cardiac performance. It is usually the radial artery pressure that is monitored, but femoral, brachial, or aortic pressures may be used.

Central venous pressure monitoring is used as an index of ventricular filling or preload; though it is truly only an index of right ventricular preload, decisions about management are usually made on the assumption that it correlates closely with left atrial pressure and it is then used as an assumption for left ventricular preload as well. Interpretation of changes in arterial blood pressure is inevitably made with reference to changes in central venous pressure. A fall in arterial blood pressure with a fall in central venous pressure is an indication that volume replacement is required. Conversely, a fall in arterial blood pressure with a rise in central venous pressure is an indication that inotropic support may be required and that cardiac tamponade should be considered and excluded.

The insertion of central venous pressure lines allows rapid and reliable delivery of intravenous drugs to the circulation. Most of these lines are removed 24 to 48 hours after the patient has been transferred out of the intensive care unit, and any that remain in place for more than seven days should be changed to reduce the risk of infection, particularly septicaemia, associated with these catheters. Historically most of these catheters had only a single lumen, which meant that several catheters had to be inserted in each patient, but there is now an increasing tendency to insert a single catheter with multiple lumens instead. This is probably safer, as it requires only one hole in the appropriate vein, but it has the drawback of being more expensive than several single lumen catheters.

Pulmonary artery pressure

Swan–Ganz catheters for monitoring pulmonary artery pressure are a mainstay of invasive monitoring in intensive care units. They are not commonly used after cardiac operations in the United Kingdom, and are restricted to patients who have been identified beforehand as being at high operative risk, and those who developed unexpected difficulties on the intensive care unit. A pulmonary artery pressure catheter can not only measure pulmonary artery pressures themselves, but also the pulmonary artery capillary wedge pressure which gives an indirect assessment of left atrial pressure. The usual assumption made is that left atrial pressure is directly related to left ventricular end diastolic pressure; this is of course incorrect in the case of mitral valve disease. If it is not possible to obtain the pulmonary artery capillary wedge pressure then the pulmonary artery diastolic pressure is commonly used instead. Direct measurements of cardiac output by the thermodilution technique can be provided at intervals and indirect estimates of change in cardiac output can be provided continuously by measurements of mixed venous oxygen saturation. Pulmonary artery catheters are also necessary if one wishes to manipulate pulmonary vascular resistance—for example, after mitral valve surgery or cardiac transplantation (see fig 4.1).

Left atrial pressure

In much the same way as it is possible to measure pressures from the right atrium or superior vena cava at operation through catheters placed percutaneously by the anaesthetist, it is relatively easy for the surgeon to measure left atrial pressures. A catheter is placed directly into the left atrium, either by cannulating the right superior pulmonary vein and passing the catheter into the body of the left atrium, or by passing a cannula through the right atrial purse string and then across the interatrial septum so that its tip lies in the left atrium. Both these approaches allow the catheters to be brought out through the skin along the chest wall and they can be withdrawn later without reopening the chest.

It is occasionally necessary to site catheters in either the pulmonary artery or the ascending aorta, but the sternotomy often has to be reopened to remove them.

27

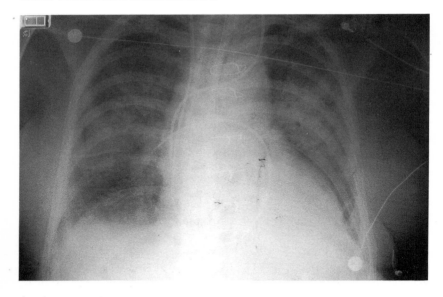

Figure 4.1 Pulmonary artery (Swan-Ganz) catheter in position. The pulmonary artery catheter is seen passing through the superior vena cava, right atrium, and right ventricle, and then passing in a gentle curve into the right pulmonary artery. Note also the sternal wires, as this patient had had coronary artery surgery.

Blood gases and electrolytes

Serial monitoring of blood gases is a considerable part of the work load. The PaO_2 is used to guide manipulations of the inspired oxygen concentration and the $PaCO_2$ is used to guide manipulations of the respiratory rate and volume. Failure of abnormal blood gases to improve after simple manoeuvres such as physiotherapy will require special treatment, such as positive end expiratory pressure (PEEP), in a ventilated patient, or continuous positive airway pressure (CPAP) in a patient who is not being ventilated.

The pH and base excess are measured from the blood gases, and a lowering of pH and an increasingly negative base excess indicate worsening tissue perfusion. This is best treated initially by measures that directly improve cardiac output. Monitoring of the potassium concentration is of considerable importance, because a low concentration increases the risk of tachyarrhythmias and a raised concentration could cause cardiac asystole. Generally, though not always, the serum concentration of potassium reflects the urine

---

Respiratory variables monitored

- Respiratory rate
- Tidal volume
- Inspired oxygen concentration
- End tidal carbon dioxide
- Pulse oximetry
- Blood gases

---

output, the serum potassium tending to fall in those patients with a copious urine output and remaining raised in those with a poor urine output.

Renal function

A urinary catheter is inserted at the time of induction of anaesthesia to allow urine output to be measured. Renal function as measured by urine output is the best indirect assessment of cardiac output, short of actually measuring cardiac output with a thermodilution catheter. The use of diuretics, plasma expanders, and agents such as dopamine must be considered when urine output is assessed. If a patient has a stable blood pressure, is warming up, and passing reasonable volumes of urine then he or she is making reasonable progress. A reduction in urine output that does not respond to simple measures is a cause for concern and an indication for further investigation. This would indicate that a pulmonary artery catheter should be inserted if one has not previously been placed. A urine output of about 0·5 ml/kg/hour is usually considered to be adequate, though in the early period after bypass it is common to see a considerably higher urine output.

It is usual to leave the urinary catheter in place until an adequate diuresis has been established. It is safer to remove the catheter first thing in the

---

Renal and metabolic variables monitored

- Temperature
- Urine output
- Acid base and base excess
- Urea and creatinine
- Mixed venous oxygen saturation

---

morning or last thing at night, because it is much easier to treat the occasional patient who goes into acute retention six or eight hours after the catheter has been removed if it happens at a relatively convenient time. The move towards silastic coated catheters, and a reduction in the time for which they are left in place has resulted in a reduction in the number of late postoperative urethral strictures. This used to be a common late complication.

Temperature

Manipulation of body temperature has played an important part in cardiac surgery from the earliest days when it was used to permit closure of atrial septal defects without cardiopulmonary bypass. The patient was cooled in an ice bath down to 30°C, and then rewarmed in water baths afterwards. In modern practice, most patients are electively cooled to temperatures of between 26 and 31°C during the operation. In paediatric surgery and some forms of aortic surgery in adults patients are cooled to temperatures as low as 15°C. The body temperature is lowered either to assist in preserving the heart from the effects of ischaemia, or (at the much lower temperatures) to allow the circulation to be completely interrupted for periods of up to 40 minutes without causing serious cerebral damage. Although the patients will be fully rewarmed on cardiopulmonary bypass, it is usual for them to cool off again in the hour or so between the end of bypass and their arrival in the intensive care unit. This will happen to any patient undergoing a major operation, and monitoring of the progress towards returning to their normal body temperature is an important element of their care. An unusually slow rise in central temperature, or persistence of a temperature gradient down the legs is suggestive of poor cardiac output and measures such as transfusion of colloid fluids and giving vasodilators and inotropes should be considered.

Analgesia

During the first 48 hours opiates are used for analgesia, usually morphine and papavaretum (Omnopon), particularly now that noscopine has been removed from the latter compound. Papavaretum is a mixture of opium alkaloids with a pharmacological structure similar to that of morphine. Through its actions on the brain it induces a state of relaxation and euphoria, together with a moderate hypnotic effect. A serious side effect in this group of drugs is their propensity to depress respiration by reducing sensitivity to increases in $PaCO_2$. They can also cause nausea (from delayed gastric emptying) and constipation (from direct effects on smooth muscle of the gut). Hypotension and bradycardia may also develop, and these usually respond to appropriate volume replacement. Morphine itself can be used in a similar way to papavaretum, as can synthetic agents such as buprenorphine. Fentanyl and alfentanyl are reserved for patients who are being ventilated. There has been increasing interest in the use of continuous intravenous opiate

---

Other variables monitored

- Blood glucose concentration
- Analgesia
  Opiates
  Paracetamol
  Prostaglandin antagonists
- Drains and drainage

---

infusions, and this is now progressing to the use of patient controlled analgesic devices.

About 48 to 72 hours after operation compound preparations of the less potent synthetic opiates together with paracetamol are usually introduced and patients will continue to take these well into the convalescent period. A typical such agent is codydramol, a combination of 10 mg dihydrocodeine tartrate and 500 mg paracetamol. In due course pain will be controlled by paracetamol alone, and eventually patients will no longer need analgesia.

Prostaglandin antagonists such as diclofenac have attracted considerable interest in postoperative analgesia, but their use has been restricted by concern about their effects on renal blood flow; the possibility of acute renal failure after their use for postoperative pain relief in cardiac surgery has caused some units not to use them. An additional effect that is occasionally of concern to the cardiac surgeon is that (like aspirin) they can inhibit platelet aggregation. It is, however, unusual for patients to be given them preoperatively.

Blood glucose monitoring

Blood glucose concentrations are monitored regularly after cardiac surgery, as they are in any intensive care unit, as part of the metabolic assessment of the patient. Apart from in diabetic patients, blood glucose concentrations are commonly raised in patients who need adrenaline infusions, and after cardiac transplantation as a result of the immunosuppressive doses of steroids. Management is by titrated infusions of insulin, together with appropriate regimens of crystalloid and colloid replacement.

Drains

Two or more drainage tubes are usually inserted at the end of the operation, which allow the blood that inevitably collects within the pericardial space after the operation to drain freely and avoid cardiac compression or tamponade. One drain is placed in the anterior mediastinum, the pericardium being left open at the end of the operation. A second drain is sited

31

behind the heart in the pericardial cavity and if the pleura has been opened a further drain will be placed in the pleural space. The drains also allow the rate of bleeding to be monitored. The classic error is to assume that a sudden reduction in drainage means that the bleeding has stopped, but particularly if the patient's haemodynamic state deteriorates the possibility that the drains have blocked must be considered. The drains are closed systems connected to a vacuum source, and they remain in place until the hourly loss has reached an acceptably low figure, usually less than 10 or 20 ml blood for two or three consecutive hours.

Common problems and special measures after cardiac surgery

Bleeding and blood transfusion

The indications for blood transfusion in cardiac surgery are changing, and there are strong moves in most centres to reduce the amount of blood used. First of all there must be meticulous attention to surgical technique, with increased emphasis on preventing bleeding on the way into the chest, and before the heparin is reversed with protamine. Any blood that is shed when the patient is not heparinised is lost, as it cannot be recirculated through the cardiopulmonary bypass pump. Some units have cell savers, but the routine use of these expensive machines has to be balanced against the improvements that can be gained simply through attention to surgical technique.

The elective removal of 500 ml of blood during the period before heparin is given, and its replacement with a synthetic plasma expander allows the patient to be mildly haemodiluted before bypass, and provides a unit of fresh blood for transfusion at the end of the operation. The bypass circuitry should be flushed through to allow a further unit of blood to be transfused at the end of the operation. It is accepted that this has a much lower haemoglobin content than the patient had at the start of the operation, because of the diluting effects of the clear fluid prime used for the bypass circuit. If one accepts a normovolaemic anaemia the pressure to transfuse a patient is reduced. Because of the lack of evidence that routinely transfusing blood into a cardiac surgical patient to an arbitrary haemoglobin concentration has any particular benefit, many units are coming to accept lower early postoperative haemoglobin concentrations providing that the patient is not hypovolaemic. Patients have a diuresis during the postoperative period and the haemoglobin concentration will increase considerably before discharge.

Autologous transfusion

Another technique used to avoid homologous transfusion is pre-donation of blood by the patient for use during the operation. The main limitation to its use has been the reluctance of blood transfusion units to set up systems whereby autologous blood can be used, because it requires the same standards of documentation as conventional homologous blood. Patients are required to donate two or more units of their own blood at intervals of a week, finishing a week before their planned operation date. It is necessary for patients to be given operation dates well in advance so that urgent and emergency cases can be added to the lists without appreciably delaying the patients who have pre-donated autologous bloods.

Homologous transfusion

For most fit adult patients with uncomplicated disease, the indications for bank blood transfusion then become either a haemoglobin concentration below an arbitrary level — say 0.08 g/l (8.0 mg/dl), or continuing and appreciable blood loss. In current practice blood is usually transfused as packed red cells resuspended in isotonic transport medium. This allows the platelets, white cells, and plasma fractions to be removed in the blood transfusion laboratories and used as isolated blood components. Some of these components are used in cardiac surgery, both platelets and clotting components being transfused under certain circumstances.

Fresh frozen plasma is indicated for patients who bleed excessively after sternotomy and who are known to have an abnormality of coagulation, usually a prolonged prothrombin time. Cryoprecipitate is indicated for transfusion into patients who are bleeding excessively, and who have a deficiency of circulating fibrinogen.

The transfusion of platelets is indicated in patients who are bleeding excessively and in whom the platelet count is depressed. Platelet numbers are commonly depressed after cardiopulmonary bypass, as a result of dilution, of platelet activation, and of consumption on the surfaces of the tubing used for the cardiopulmonary bypass circuit. Furthermore, platelet function is irreversibly depressed in patients who have been taking aspirin within a week of operation. As a result of this the use of platelets tends to be higher in the unstable patients who are having urgent or emergency operations.

Other methods to limit the need for blood transfusion

Apart from autologous blood transfusion and the flushing through of the bypass circuit there are mechanical and pharmacological ways of reducing blood loss. The first mechanical method is meticulous surgical technique, though this should go without saying. The next method is the use of cell saver machines by which shed blood is aspirated from the operative field. It is centrifuged to remove debris and other cellular fragments from the red cells which are then resuspended in normal saline for transfusion.

The first pharmacological method of blood conservation is to reverse the heparin with protamine after the operation. Enough protamine should be used to return the activated clotting time to its control value. Agents such as tranexamic acid have proved to be disappointing in the prevention of bleeding after cardiopulmonary bypass, though there is some suggestion that

---

Common early problems after cardiac operations

- Bleeding
- Haemodynamic instability
- Respiratory failure
- Arrhythmias

- Bradyarrhythmias
- Low cardiac output
- Low urinary output

---

they are of use when given after the operation. There is, however, clear evidence of benefit from the prophylactic use of high dose aprotinin given during the operation. The exact mechanism of action remains uncertain, and it is generally reserved for patients having reoperations or other high risk procedures, though there is an increasing tendency to use it during more routine cases.

Airway management in the early postoperative period

Patients remain intubated until they are haemodynamically stable, not bleeding, awake or rousable, able to maintain their own airway, and able to achieve satisfactory ventilatory measurements. These criteria in the early postoperative period would be a PaO_2 greater than 10 kPa, a $PaCO_2$ less than 5.5 kPa on less than 50% fractional inspired oxygen (FiO_2). The length of time taken to achieve extubation varies from unit to unit according to the anaesthetic and postoperative management protocols in use.

Prolonged postoperative ventilation

Ventilation is indicated in patients who are haemodynamically unstable, bleeding during the postoperative period or who have a degree of respiratory failure. In the latter group the problem will be either failure to oxygenate, failure to excrete carbon dioxide, or a combination of the two. This is generally seen together with sepsis, prolonged low cardiac output, or multiple system organ failure.

Treatment of respiratory dysfunction

Treatments range from the simple manoeuvres of physiotherapy and supplying oxygen by face mask to increase the FiO2, through facial continuous positive airway pressure (facial CPAP) by mask, to continued intubation, or reintubation, and the use of various different ventilatory

---

Less common problems after cardiac operations

- Damage to central nervous system
- Damage to other organs
- Multiple system organ failure

---

modes. Antiasthma treatment is used if the patient has a wheeze, and on rare occasions respiratory stimulants such as doxapram are indicated. Minitracheostomy for suction of the airways in an extubated patient, and formal tracheostomy for weaning of an intubated patient, are useful techniques.

Minitracheostomy (cricothyroidotomy)

A minitracheostomy, more accurately named a cricothyroidotomy, is the formation of a pathway into the trachea through the cricothyroid membrane and through which the patient can undergo tracheal suction for retention of sputum. The technique was originally developed by inserting cut down neonatal endotracheal tubes through a stab wound in the cricothyroid membrane, but specially designed minitracheostomy kits are now available.

The procedure is indicated in extubated patients with retention of sputum who have difficulty, even with extensive amounts of physiotherapy, in expectorating effectively. The technique was pioneered in thoracic surgery, but its application extends to all branches of medicine. It has also been used to assist ventilation, as it is possible to ventilate by jet through a minitracheostomy. The technique has also been used to gain access to the airway in an emergency, and though it is by no means ideal, it can allow enough oxygenation to be life saving.

It is contraindicated in patients with bleeding disorders as the most common major complication is haemorrhage from the site of insertion. The main risk is of bleeding into the trachea, though this can generally be managed with pressure around the point of entry and repeated tracheal suction through the minitracheostomy itself.

The procedure is done under local anaesthesia and the cricothyroid membrane is identified below the laryngeal prominence and above the cricoid ring by its usually elastic texture. After the area has been cleaned and draped, local anaesthetic is infiltrated into the skin and overlying soft tissues, and then through the cricothyroid membrane itself and into the trachea. A stab incision is made through the skin and cricothyroid membrane and into the trachea. This is much easier if patients can be persuaded to hold their breath for a few moments. An introducer is guided into the trachea through the incision, and the minitracheostomy itself is inserted over the introducer. The minitracheostomy is secured with tapes after tracheal suction (fig 4.2).

The minitracheostomy is not removed until the patient is able to cough and

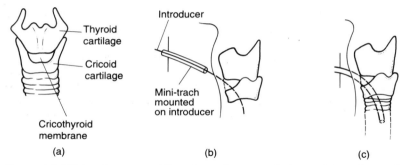

Figure 4.2 Minitracheostomy. The minitracheostomy is inserted into the trachea through a stab incision in the cricothyroid membrane.

protect their airway. The tube is taken out and an occlusive dressing placed over the stoma in the neck, which rapidly closes.

Tracheostomy

Tracheostomy is indicated for maintenance of the airway when orotracheal or nasotracheal intubation is inappropriate. Apart from the emergency indications for tracheostomy, which are not relevant here, it is most commonly used as part of the process of weaning sick patients off long term ventilation (usually longer than two weeks). These patients often need to be awake with minimal sedation, and in these conditions they are often intolerant of standard endotracheal intubation. Tracheostomy for these patients significantly improves their comfort and allows them to be ventilated, and weaned from their ventilation, whilst they are awake. In addition it lowers the work of breathing.

Insertion of a tracheostomy

The standard technique for insertion of a tracheostomy tube is by a surgical cut down. Though the operation can be done in the intensive care unit, there is little doubt that it is technically easier in an operating theatre on an operating table. The patient's neck is gently extended on a head ring with a sand bag under the shoulders, and a skin crease incision of about 3 cm in length is made about 1 cm above the sternal notch. The fascia is divided and the strap muscles separated to expose the front of the trachea. It is sometimes necessary to divide the isthmus of the thyroid gland, though usually it can just be retracted. Having placed stay sutures in the trachea, and checked that the tracheostomy tube is of the right size and that the appropriate connectors fit, a vertical incision is made through the second and third tracheal rings and the tracheostomy tube inserted. The tube is secured with tapes after tracheal suction, and the skin edges loosely approximated with one or two interrupted sutures on each side of the tube.

There are various types of tracheostomy tubes, the most common ones having high volume low pressure cuffs, this configuration being chosen to minimise the risks of tracheal necrosis from long term intubation.

The tracheostomy is removed when the patient is able to cough and protect the airway, in addition to having adequate blood gas tensions on a low inspired oxygen concentration. The tube is taken out and an occlusive dressing placed over the stoma in the neck which rapidly closes over. Occasionally a minitracheostomy is inserted to prevent the stoma closing immediately.

Arrhythmias

Tachyarrhythmias

Both ventricular and supraventricular tachyarrhythmias can occur after cardiac surgery. Ventricular ectopics occur, but usually settle if an adequate serum potassium concentration is maintained. If they become frequent they warrant further treatment, and lignocaine is the drug of choice.

Ventricular tachycardia (VT) and ventricular fibrillation (VF) are both uncommon, but if they do develop after operation the likelihood is of operative myocardial damage or ongoing myocardial ischaemia. Assuming that the arterial blood gases and serum potassium concentration are in the appropriate range, ventricular tachycardia should be treated with either lignocaine (1 mg/kg slow bolus) or DC cardioversion, as appropriate. A lignocaine infusion, starting at 3–4 mg/minute and decreasing if no further VT occurred, would then be appropriate. Ventricular fibrillation requires immediate DC cardioversion, and should then be followed by loading with lignocaine and a lignocaine infusion. A careful study of the serial ECGs should be made for evidence of ischaemia and any abnormalities of the arterial blood gases or serum potassium quickly corrected.

Atrial tachyarrhythmias are more common, and develop in up to 10% of patients postoperatively. They are rarely more than a nuisance, and in the first instance the arterial blood gases and serum potassium concentration should be checked and the appropriate corrections made. An intravenous loading dose of amiodarone is our first line of treatment and is usually followed by rapid reversion to sinus rhythm. The standard loading dose is 300 mg over one hour followed by 900 mg over the next 24 hours, and this should be enough to convert the patient back into sinus rhythm. A short oral course of amiodarone should then be given, and this may be stopped before the patient is discharged. Amiodarone should be given for more than 6 weeks only under the direction of a cardiologist. Digoxin is no longer used as a first line of treatment.

The evidence for prophylaxis against atrial arrhythmias after cardiac surgery shows little signs of benefit and we do not use prophylactic antiarrhythmic drugs.

Bradyarrhythmias: Pacing

Temporary pacing of the heart can be required after cardiac surgery, particularly when cardioplegia has been used for myocardial preservation. It is also more common after valve operations than after those on the coronary arteries.

Pacing is indicated when the ventricular rate is slower than optimum. Obviously if stroke volume is relatively fixed, or is already maximised by judicious volume loading, then cardiac output is dependent on heart rate and the afterload. The mode of pacing is governed by the underlying cardiac rhythm; if the rhythm is a sinus bradycardia then the most appropriate pacing mode is atrial pacing, and similarly for nodal rhythm. Complete heart block is best treated with sequential atrial and ventricular pacing, and ventricular pacing alone should be reserved for atrial fibrillation where there is a slow ventricular rate. Pacing is also used in the treatment of some arrhythmias, to overdrive the heart and thereby attempt to break the reentry circuit.

Temporary epicardial pacing wires are easily inserted at operation, simply by sewing ventricular wires directly into the myocardium or by sewing atrial wires to the atrium with fine stitches. The wires are then brought out through the skin to the surface to be connected to temporary pacing boxes. In both

---

Pacemaker code

Position in code	Meaning	Abbreviations
I	Chamber(s) paced	V Ventricle
		A Atrium
		D Double
II	Chamber(s) sensed	V Ventricle
		A Atrium
		D Double
		O None
III	Mode of response	T Trigger
		I Inhibit
		D Double
		O None
		R Reverse
IV	Programmable functions	P Programmable rate and/or output
		M Multi-programmable
V	Special tachyarrhythmia functions	B Burst
		N Normal rate competition
		S Scanning
		E External

cases the wires can be pulled out when they are no longer required. It is traditional, but probably unnecessary, to document that the international normalised ratio is below 2 before they are removed. With a ventricular pacing system alone the pacing box should be set to a demand mode, to avoid an electrical "R on T" event with its consequent risks of ventricular arrhythmias. With many of the less sophisticated temporary pacing boxes it is not possible to use a demand mode for atrial pacing and so a fixed rate mode is used. Sequential atrioventricular pacing requires sophisticated pacing boxes that can provide the full range of dual chamber pacing modes. It is usual for temporary epicardial ventricular pacing wires to have an initial threshold of less than one volt, whereas it is common for atrial epicardial pacing wires to have a threshold of three volts or more.

Low cardiac output

Cardiac output may be low initially, and is indicated by cool peripheries with a failure to warm, normal to low arterial blood pressure, and a sluggish urine output soon after operation. Metabolic acidosis (or at least an increasingly negative base excess) reflects impaired tissue perfusion and is a common coexisting feature. Measurement of the central venous pressure is the initial guide to management: if it is low then the patient is probably hypovolaemic and appropriate colloid replacement should be given. If the central venous pressure is in the normal range then a transfusion of colloid can be given cautiously and the variables reassessed. If this does not produce improvement in the signs of low cardiac output, or if the central venous pressure is already raised, the introduction of inotropes should be considered. Under appropriate circumstances judicious use of vasodilators can also be helpful.

Failure to respond to low doses of inotropes, particularly if the low cardiac output was unexpected, is an indication for the insertion of a pulmonary artery pressure catheter. As indicated earlier this provides data on pulmonary artery pressures, an estimate of left atrial pressures, and a measure of cardiac output. These data can then be used as a guide to the management of the circulation. If the appropriate inotropes do not ameliorate the patient's condition then mechanical support of the failing heart must be considered. The most commonly used equipment is the intra-aortic balloon pump, and this is considered in more detail in chapter 8. Briefly it is a balloon that is placed into the descending aorta percutaneously from the femoral artery. It increases coronary artery blood flow in diastole by inflating as the aortic valve closes and reduces afterload by deflating in presystole.

If the balloon pump fails to maintain the circulation in combination with the appropriate inotropes, then a ventricular assist device can be inserted. These devices vary in their availability and effectiveness, and are discussed in more detail in chapter 8.

Low urine output

Renal failure is a serious cause of morbidity after cardiac surgery, though fortunately it is usually reversible after a suitable period of support. Some patients are at higher risk of developing renal failure, particularly those with pre-existing renal failure, and those with sepsis or cardiogenic shock either before or after surgery. There are two complementary approaches to the management of renal failure: the first is to avoid its onset, and the second is to support the patient effectively if this fails.

Avoidance of renal failure starts by ensuring that the patient is adequately hydrated before operation, and that the circulating blood volume is adequate after operation. Nephrotoxic agents (including the aminoglycoside antibiotics such as gentamicin) should be used with caution and their concentration monitored to ensure that adequate but not excessive doses are used. It is also becoming common to run a so-called "renal" dose of dopamine before, during, and after cardiopulmonary bypass in patients thought to be at risk of renal failure.

The standard criterion for an acceptable urine output in the early postoperative period is generally considered to be 0.5 ml/kg/minute. If this target is not achieved then various measures may be undertaken. Firstly the patient is given a volume load big enough to ensure adequate central venous and systemic pressures. If this is achieved without improvement in urine flow then a low dose of dopamine should be started, usually about 2 μg/kg/ minute. After this, loop diuretics should be given, starting with a low dose of frusemide such as 20 mg intravenously, but increased as appropriate. If this strategy is unsuccessful then more invasive forms of renal support should be considered.

Renal support after cardiac surgery

Renal support is indicated when simple methods to ensure adequate urine output (including appropriate volume loading, dopamine and diuretics) have failed, and the patient has increasing acidosis and hyperkalaemia. The usual indication will be a serum potassium concentration above 6.0 mmol/l and rising in conjunction with a urine output of considerably less than 0.5 ml/kg/ hour after treatment.

There are various ways of supplying renal support; conventional haemo-dialysis is not usually used in the early postoperative period as it may cause appreciable haemodynamic instability. The most common techniques are haemofiltration or haemodiafiltration. In haemofiltration the blood is passed through a filter to produce an ultrafiltrate. The amount of volume lost is then replaced with a physiological balanced salt solution, such as Hartmann's. In haemodiafiltration the technique is modified slightly so that an electrolyte solution is run in a counter current direction to the blood stream across the

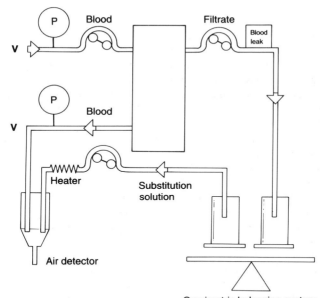

Figure 4.3 Automatic haemofiltration pump.

membrane of the filter. This allows both the removal of fluid by ultrafiltration and also the dialysis of permeable molecules across the membrane down the concentration gradient.

Both techniques can be run as either arteriovenous or venovenous shunts. In the former the pressure of blood from a large artery is used to push the blood through the filter and then into a large vein, and in the latter blood is pumped from a large vein through the filter by a small pump, before being returned into the same vein or another large vein (see fig 4.3). This venovenous route has the considerable advantage that blood can be removed from and returned to the same vein with a double lumen catheter. This avoids the need for arterial cannulation with its consequent risks.

Other complications after cardiac surgery

Central nervous system damage

The incidence of discrete central nervous system damage or stroke is consistently about 2% after coronary surgery. It is age related, increasing from 0.5% for patients in their fifties to 5% in patients over 70 years of age. The commonest cause is probably embolisation of atherosclerotic debris from the ascending aorta. Some affected patients have had previous transient

41

Tracheostomy

- Indicated for:
  Sputum retention
  Increased ventilation
  Access to airway
- Contraindicated if the patient is bleeding

---

ischaemic attacks, but the presence of asymptomatic carotid artery disease is not predictive. Most cases are relatively mild and recover, but a few have persisting severe disability. Stroke is sufficiently common, and the consequences so serious, that the risk must be specifically mentioned before operation to both the patient and the family. The incidence of stroke is higher in valve patients as these will have had their hearts opened, and there is the risk of embolisation of air as well as particulate debris.

Diffuse cerebral injury that alters short term memory and concentration is common, but is only discernible by comparing carefully performed neuropsychological tests before and after operation. It can then be identified in a third of patients two months after operation, and is still present at a year. Subjective complaints are a poor guide to the presence of this form of cortical damage, and complaints of cognitive deficit correlate more with depressed mood state than with objective evidence of neuropsychological deterioration.

Damage to other organs

Cardiopulmonary bypass and major cardiac surgery are associated with damage to other organs including lung, kidneys, and gastrointestinal tract. These are more common the longer the bypass time, the more severe the disease, and the older the patient. They are rare in routine elective cases. Isolated coronary surgery rarely leads to multiple system organ failure.

The future

The main future developments in postoperative cardiac surgical intensive care are expected to be manipulations to reduce the time that a patient stays on the intensive care unit, and these will develop from efforts to improve the condition in which patients are presented to the intensive care unit. A side effect of this will be an increase in the numbers of patients who never go to an intensive care unit but are transferred directly to a high dependency unit. In practical terms most high dependency units are able to fulfil all the features of an intensive care unit except ventilation. Some high dependency units are able to carry out techniques such as haemofiltration and intra-aortic balloon pumping together with other techniques such as providing facial or nasal continuous positive airway pressure for respiratory support.

Another major change is the increasing use of microprocessors for transferring data from monitoring equipment, as well as directly from ventilators and infusion pumps. This vastly reduces the workload required to maintain accurate records of postoperative events. In the near future this has the potential to abolish the use of paper charts for data recording, which will also allow data to be presented in more convenient forms for both research and audit. A further potential is that it allows quick and accurate transmission of data to and from other sites, so that, for instance, a patient's behaviour in the operating theatre can be monitored on the intensive care unit and vice versa.

5 Surgery for coronary artery disease

- Selection of patients
- Indications for operation to relieve symptoms
- Indications for operation to improve prognosis
- Coronary bypass operation
- Cardiac operation
- Mortality and morbidity
- Outlook after coronary artery surgery
- Appendix: anatomy of coronary arteries

Selection of patients likely to benefit

Operations on the coronary arteries make up most of the workload in a western cardiac surgical unit, and over the years clear indications for such operations have been laid down. Surgical intervention is aimed at both the relief of symptoms and the reduction of the risk of premature death. Surgical revascularisation of the myocardium by bypass grafting is effective in achieving both goals, and in most patients both objectives play a part in the decision to operate.

As an indication of the volume of work undertaken, in the United Kingdom a target of 300 operations/million head of population/year was suggested at a consensus conference in London in 1984. This figure was accepted by the Department of Health in 1986, although most cardiologists and cardiac surgeons now think that this figure is too low. The figures for 1990 are shown in the box. What is also clear about practice in the United Kingdom is that neighbouring districts in the same region can have enormous

---

Coronary artery bypass grafts

	Number/million, 1990
United Kingdom	278 (regional range 97–466)
Australia	700
United States	1800

---

variations in operative rates, and this probably reflects both the geographical relation to cardiac surgical centres, as well as the attitudes of the referring physicians and the commissioning agencies.

When considering the management of patients with coronary artery disease, it is worth considering symptoms and prognosis separately at the decision making stage, as there are two questions to be asked:

- Would operation be justified just to relieve the patient's symptoms?
- Would operation be expected to prolong the patient's survival, given the particular pattern of coronary artery disease?

If the answer to either question is "yes", then operation is indicated; commonly it is justified on both grounds. As experience with cardiac surgery increases, and as specialist cardiologists become more widely available, it is clear that many patients who were not previously considered for operation should now be. It is much better for a few patients to have unnecessary exercise tests than for others not to be investigated for angina and subsequently infarct before they have a cardiological assessment.

The final decision on the management of ischaemic heart disease includes technical considerations, and depends on the results of investigations which always include a coronary angiogram, usually an exercise test, and sometimes one or more nuclear test. The severity and exact nature of the symptoms are, however, central to this part of the decision making process. The history must be reviewed by the surgeon in the light of the data provided by the investigations.

History

The interview must focus on the severity of symptoms, the extent to which they are attributable to reversible myocardial ischaemia, and whether adequate attempts have been made to relieve them by medical treatment. It is important to assess the extent to which the patient will benefit from the relief of angina. If other disease or handicap limits mobility and subjective wellbeing, then relief of exercise–induced angina may make little contribution to health or the enjoyment of life. On the other hand, angina severe enough to interfere with a reasonable amount of activity while on appropriate medical treatment is clearly sufficient indication to consider operation.

Risk factors should be reviewed, because if they continue unchecked they will reduce the benefit obtained from operation. Those that can be influenced include smoking, diabetes, hypertension, hyperlipidaemia, obesity, and diet. Family history cannot be changed, but it is an opportunity to advise the family to reduce the risks for the next generation. Of particular interest to the risk-benefit analysis is a history of transient ischaemic attacks or stroke. Clearly in the elective patients it is possible to try and make changes in risk factors, though it is impossible in those who are unstable. Obese patients can help the mechanics of their breathing by losing weight, and this also reduces the energy demand on an ischaemic heart. People who are smoking at the time of operation seem to stay in hospital longer and develop more chest and sternal wound complications.

Clinical examination

Availability and suitability of the long saphenous vein should be established. Varicosity or surgical removal of the saphenous system does not preclude coronary bypass surgery, but it may make revascularisation more difficult to achieve and less predictable in its outcome. If that is the case a careful assessment of the short saphenous veins and the veins of the arms should be made. The general suitability of the patient to undergo a major operation, particularly with reference to renal function, should be assessed at the same time.

Specific investigations

Every patient will have had a coronary angiogram and the films will usually have been reviewed by the surgeon before he sees the patient. The anatomical extent of the coronary artery disease, including the site and severity of the stenoses, is a major determinant of prognosis. In a patient with angina or evidence of silent ischaemia, the more proximal the stenoses, and the more vessels involved, the worse the outlook without treatment. On the other hand, these patients will receive relatively greater benefit from surgical revascularisation than patients with a small number of relatively distal stenoses. There is clear evidence of improved survival in patients operated on for left main stem and triple–vessel coronary artery disease. There is no evidence of improved survival for single or double–vessel coronary artery disease, although a lesion of the proximal left anterior descending coronary artery is still (for most people) worrying. This evidence is based on relatively old data, however, and there have certainly been technical improvements in coronary artery surgery since then, particularly in the increasing use of arterial grafts that would be expected to improve the benefit of surgery and lessen its risk. Figure 5.1 shows normal coronary angiogram; figures 5.2, 5.3, and 5.4 show variants of coronary artery disease.

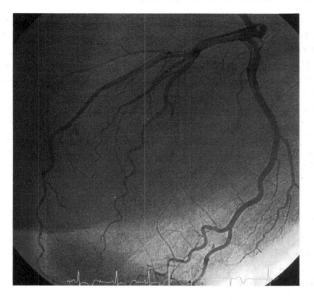

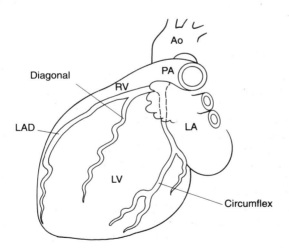

Figure 5.1 Normal coronary arteries as seen angiographically and a view of the heart in the same projection.

a. Left coronary artery and left lateral view of the heart.

Ao: aorta, LV: left ventricle, RV: right ventricle, RA: right atrium, LA: left atrium, PA: pulmonary artery, SVC: superior vena cava, LAD: left anterior descending or anterior interventricular coronary artery.

47

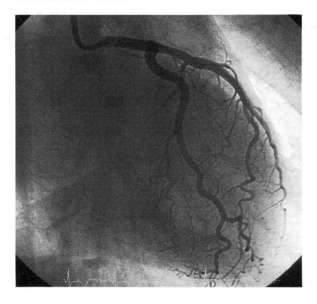

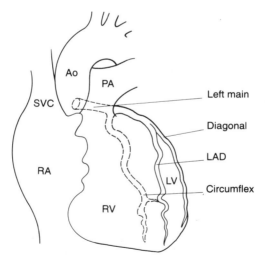

Figure 5.1 Normal coronary arteries as seen angiographically and a view of the heart in the same projection.
b. Left coronary artery and anterior view of the heart, a little to the right.
Ao: aorta, LV: left ventricle, RV: right ventricle, RA: right atrium, LA: left atrium, PA: pulmonary artery, SVC: superior vena cava, LAD: left anterior descending or anterior interventricular coronary artery.

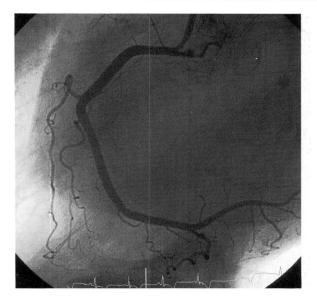

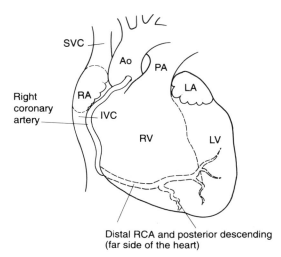

Figure 5.1 Normal coronary arteries as seen angiographically and a view of the heart in the same projection.
c. Right coronary artery and an anterior view of the heart
Ao: aorta, LV: left ventricle, RV: right ventricle, RA: right atrium, LA: left atrium, PA: pulmonary artery, SVC: superior vena cava, LAD: left anterior descending or anterior interventricular coronary artery.

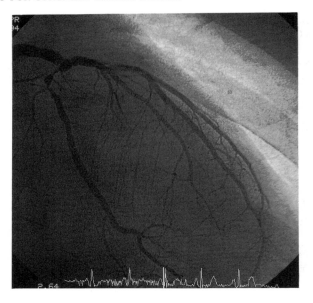

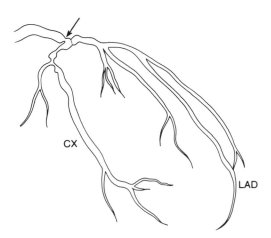

Figure 5.2 Left coronary angiogram in the right anterior oblique projection showing the left anterior descending coronary artery (LAD) with its diagonal branches, and the circumflex system (Cx). There are obvious severe narrowings in the proximal circumflex artery, but also there is a severe narrowing in the distal left main coronary artery (arrowed).

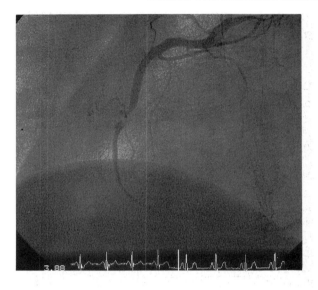

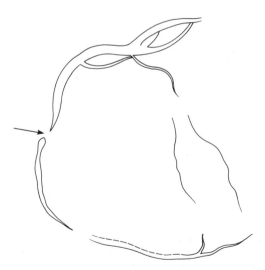

Figure 5.3 The right coronary artery is blocked (arrowed). The vessels can be seen to fill as a ghost through collaterals.

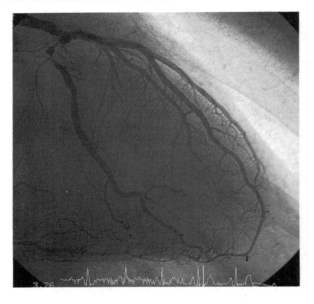

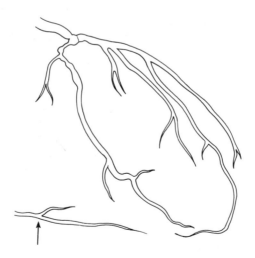

Figure 5.4 The left coronary artery is seen as in 5.1 but now the posterior descending coronary artery (arrowed), the terminal portion of the blocked right coronary artery, can be seen filling through collaterals.

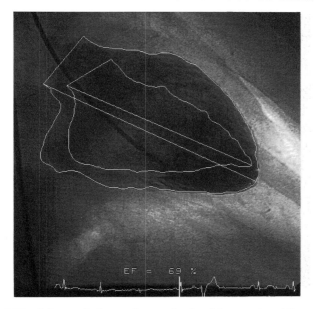

Figure 5.5 The left ventricular angiogram in the right anterior oblique projection with the end systolic end the diastolic contours outlined.

The state of the left ventricle is important in defining prognosis and it may be judged by left ventricular cine angiography (fig. 5.5), echocardiography or gated acquisition nuclear ventriculography. The poorer the left ventricular function, the worse the natural history, and conversely the greater the margin of benefit in terms of survival after surgical revascularisation compared with medical management.

If there is doubt about the attribution of symptoms to myocardial ischaemia, or a need for objective evaluation of their severity, a graded exercise test with continuous measurement of the electrocardiogram should be done at this stage if it has not already been done. Myocardial perfusion scintigrams may help in difficult cases to decide if there is an area of reversible ischaemia where a coronary bypass graft would be of use. This is sometimes helpful in assessing the need for repeat operation.

Indications for operation to relieve symptoms

Coronary artery bypass grafting is a highly effective way to relieve angina. The subjective sensations of tightness, choking, heaviness, or even "breathlessness" may all be signs of ischaemia, and can all be relieved by revascularisation. Pain alone is often not described and may even be denied by the patient. Atypical symptoms, provided that there is convincing evidence that they are caused by myocardial ischaemia, are just as likely to be relieved.

Operation to relieve angina should be considered for any patient who has a reasonable expectation of activity or enjoyment of life curtailed by angina despite an adequate trial of medical treatment. The threshold at which operation is considered for symptoms will vary according to a realistic estimate of the risks of death and morbidity for the individual patient. The likelihood of leaving hospital alive is 97%, a figure which has been stable for a number of years according to the United Kingdom Cardiac Surgery Register, and will therefore apply to the average case; typically male, aged 55 to 65, with triple–vessel coronary artery disease, and no worse than "moderate" impairment of left ventricular function. The estimate should be adjusted up or down according to the risk factors for the individual patient. It will also have to be modified as time goes by, depending on the available resources and success of medical treatment or angioplasty. In practice well over 90% of patients are free of angina at one year, and this benefit is maintained in 80% at five years and 60% at ten years.

Indications for operation to improve prognosis

The first step is to find out if the patient is in a category with a poor prognosis. If not, operation really cannot be justified on these grounds and the patient should be reassured that as far as one can predict the outlook is good. The important point is that a small risk of death, with an unpredictable time course, cannot predictably be reduced by a major operation with its own inherent risks. Three factors particularly associated with a poor natural history are: the anatomical distribution of coronary stenoses, impaired left ventricular function and evidence of myocardial ischaemia at low workload.

Anatomical distribution of coronary stenoses

The anatomical patterns which are particularly dangerous are left main stem stenosis, disease involving all three major vessels, and two–vessel

---

Postoperative relief from angina

	Percentage of patients
● At one year	90
● At five years	80
● At ten years	60

coronary artery disease when one of the vessels is the left anterior descending coronary artery. Coronary artery surgery improves survival in these groups of patients. The risks of death attributable to these patterns of stenoses are removed by surgical revascularisation, which restores the patient to the background risks of patients with only mild coronary artery disease.

Impaired left ventricular function

Patients with poor left ventricular function are much more likely to die during the next few years than those with good function, irrespective of other features of their ischaemic heart disease. They have less reserve and have already shown that they are at risk of myocardial infarction. Revascularisation ameliorates that risk.

Evidence of myocardial ischaemia at low workload

For patients with angina, the worse the angina, the worse the prognosis. The same is true of myocardial ischaemia shown on the exercise test, even if it is clinically silent. Presumably this is because they have vulnerable myocardium unsupported by collateral vessels. This is a paradox, because fatal myocardial infarction is at least as likely to be caused by coronary occlusion in people with no previous evidence of ischaemia; it is often caused by thrombosis developing on mild coronary lesions. Unstable angina is not in itself a reason to operate, as if it settles with medical management, whether because an unstable plaque has stabilised or collaterals have developed, the patient is returned to a relatively low risk state, essentially governed by the underlying anatomy of the coronary arteries.

The factors that adversely influence the risk of the operation itself are older age, repeat operation, obesity, diabetes, hypertension, hyperlipidaemia, renal impairment, emergency operation, emergency after angioplasty or cardiac catheterisation, and female sex.

The factors that adversely influence long term postoperative survival include failure to use the internal mammary artery as a graft to the left anterior descending coronary artery, failure to achieve adequate revascularisation, and poor left ventricular function. Apart from patients whose left ventricular function is extremely poor, for example an ejection fraction of less than 10%, the outlook is better with revascularisation than without.

In summary, the more severe and extensive the coronary artery disease the greater is the comparative benefit of operation over medical treatment. The outlook is, however, similar if the disease is less severe. The worse the left ventricular function, the greater the comparative benefit of surgical over medical management.

Coronary bypass operation

Some knowledge of the technicalities of the operation is relevant for those who refer patients for operation and supervise their care afterwards. There are several technical options which are used according to the surgeon's preference or the suitability of the patient.

Choice of grafts and their surgical preparation

Long saphenous vein

The most commonly used graft is the long saphenous (fig 5.6) vein which is taken from the inner aspect of the leg, from the ankle to the groin, at the same time as the chest is being opened and while preparations are being made for the cardiac operation. The usual technique is to cut down through the skin and subcutaneous tissues, exactly over the vein, to avoid creating flaps which may necrose from poor blood supply. The branches of the vein are tied or clipped and the vein stored briefly in heparinised blood. Careful handling

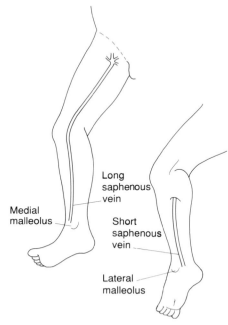

Figure 5.6 The commonest conduit used in coronary surgery is the long saphenous vein. It is long, reasonably straight, has a tolerable number of branches, is expendable and can be dissected without difficulty. The short saphenous vein is an acceptable alternative.

Risk factors for coronary artery disease

- Smoking
- Diabetes
- Hypertension
- Hyperlipidaemia
- Hypercholesterolaemia
- Obesity
- Family history

---

of the vein at this stage by avoiding high distention pressure maintains the integrity of its endothelium and perhaps long term patency. If the long saphenous vein cannot be used because of varicose disease, or because it has been stripped, one may use the short saphenous vein (which is more awkward to remove) or arm veins (which are fragile and more difficult to use).

There is no obvious difference in the results obtained with these veins. The long saphenous vein is accessible, expendable, and convenient. Vein grafts

---

Decision making in coronary surgery

Would operation be justified just to relieve the patient's symptoms?

- Operation should be considered to relieve angina when a reasonable expectation of activity or enjoyment of life is curtailed by it despite an adequate trial of medical treatment.

Would operation be expected to prolong the patient's survival, given the particular pattern of coronary artery disease?

- Particular anatomical patterns
  Left main stem stenosis
  Disease involving all three major vessels
  Two vessel coronary artery disease if one of the vessels involved is the left anterior descending coronary artery
- Impaired left ventricular function
- Evidence of myocardial ischaemia at low workload.

Age

- Not relevant

Available grafts

Veins
- Long saphenous
- Short saphenous
- Arm

Arteries
- Internal thoracic (mammary) left and right (pedicled or free)
- Right gastroepiploic
- Inferior epigastric
- Radial

Others
- Umbilical vein
- Bovine internal thoracic artery
- Bovine fetal carotid artery
- Prosthetic materials such as PTFE

almost invariably deteriorate with time. There is an early phase during the first few months when a new layer derived from platelets, fibrin, and circulating cells forms concentrically on the intimal surface and thickens the wall. The attrition rate for vein grafts is about 2% a year with a high incidence of disease in the wall and occlusion from seven years onwards. Patency at 10 years is only about 50%.

Internal mammary (thoracic) artery

Much evidence has accumulated that shows the benefits of an arterial graft with the internal mammary (thoracic) artery to the left anterior descending coronary artery both in terms of patency of the graft and survival of the patient. It is postulated that arterial grafts to other vessels might further improve the outcome after coronary artery surgery. The internal mammary artery is dissected off the chest wall with division of all its branches, but its proximal origin from the subclavian artery is left intact when possible. The artery can also be used as a free graft if necessary. The pleura is often opened during the dissection. The left internal mammary artery is used as the graft to the left anterior descending coronary artery whenever possible, the rationale being that the left anterior descending coronary artery is the most important artery in the heart, and the internal mammary artery has the best long term patency of all available grafts. Both internal mammary arteries can be used, but sternal healing may be compromised, particularly in obese and diabetic patients. Increased operating time, a second pleural opening, and more opportunity for haemorrhage all add to morbidity and may exceed any advantage gained by two internal mammary artery grafts. Double internal mammary artery grafting is an attractive option in younger patients, and evidence is gradually accumulating that it gives additional benefit compared with single internal mammary artery grafting, although currently it has not been proved. The balance of risks and benefits must be considered carefully before double internal mammary artery grafting is undertaken in older and high risk patients.

There is clear evidence that patients with a pedicled left internal mammary artery graft to the left anterior descending coronary artery are more likely to be alive, free from myocardial infarction, and free of angina, at 10 years than those with a vein graft. Patency rates at 10 years can be as good as 95%, and the artery can grow to accommodate the demands placed on it by the size of its run-off.

Other arterial grafts

Inevitably many vein grafts will fail and more patients will require repeat operation so the right gastroepiploic artery and the inferior epigastric artery have also been used. The peritoneum must be opened to harvest the right gastroepiploic artery and the artery must be dissected off the greater curvature of the stomach. It is brought up, usually anterior to the pylorus, and provides a satisfactory graft to the inferior surface of the heart. The inferior epigastric artery is used as a free conduit as, occasionally, is the radial artery.

Artificial conduits

In desperation some surgeons may turn to synthetic grafts such as those made from expanded polytetrafluoroethylene (PTFE) or to arterial tissue grafts fixed in glutaraldehyde such as fetal bovine carotid artery or bovine internal thoracic artery grafts. None has given satisfactory long term patency, though they are occasionally used when there is nothing else available.

Cardiac operation

The chest is opened through a median sternotomy, and the operation is usually done with the patient on cardiopulmonary bypass, although it is possible to do a limited operation (particularly to the left anterior descending artery and to the main right coronary artery) on a beating and working heart. The techniques of bypass and myocardial preservation are described in chapter 2.

Incomplete revascularisation is a risk factor for premature death or recurrence of angina, so all blocked or appreciably obstructed ($>50\%$) vessels that are amenable to grafting by virtue of size and quality of the wall, are grafted. Endarterectomy, when the atheroma is cored out with the intima and part of the media leaving a shell of the vessel as a conduit, is done if no better means of access to the system can be established. The distal segments of vessels in infarcted areas are grafted not only because they may be in communication with collaterals, but also because they may supply some viable myocardium and so help to relieve the ischaemia. A typical operation will include between three to five grafts.

Having instituted bypass and arrested the heart, the coronary vessels are inspected and palpated. The appropriate sites for grafting are chosen based both on the details of the coronary arteriogram and on the state of the vessels at operation. The coronary artery is usually slung between "stay" sutures at the chosen site of grafting before it is opened over a distance of 8–10 mm with a combination of scalpel and scissors. The end of the saphenous vein or internal thoracic artery is then prepared to match the incision in the coronary artery, and the two are anastomosed with a suture (fig 5.7), continuous 6.0 polypropylene (Prolene) is used for vein to coronary artery anastomoses and 7.0 polypropylene for internal thoracic artery to coronary artery anastomoses. When the anastomoses are completed the stay sutures are removed. If cardioplegia is used for myocardial protection then all the distal coronary artery anastomoses are completed first, the cross-clamp is then released from the aorta, and the proximal saphenous vein to aorta anastomoses are completed. If cross-clamp fibrillation is used for myocardial protection the

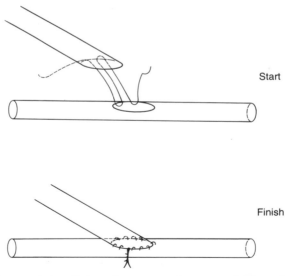

Start

Finish

Figure 5.7 In a typical technique for coronary bypass grafts the vein or internal thoracic artery is anastomosed with a continuous suture, started at the "heel" of the anastomosis, brought around the "toe" and tied mid-way down one side.

Factors that increase the risk of operation

- Older age
- Repeat operation
- Obesity
- Diabetes
- Hypertension
- Hyperlipidaemia
- Renal impairment
- Emergency operation
- Emergency after angioplasty or cardiac catheterisation
- Female sex

---

cross-clamp is released from the aorta after each distal anastomosis has been completed and the proximal anastomosis is done before the sequence is repeated. The proximal saphenous vein to aorta anastomoses are constructed with the heart being reperfused with blood after the cross-clamp has been released from the aorta. Part of the aorta is isolated by a side-biting clamp and a small hole is cut or punched in the wall of the aorta at this point. The vein graft is then measured for length after the heart has been momentarily filled with blood by temporary obstruction of the venous drainage. The end of the vein graft is prepared for anastomosis and then sutured to the aorta, usually with continuous 5.0 polypropylene. The side-biting clamp is then removed from the aorta and air removed from the vein graft. When all the coronary artery bypass grafts have been completed, the patient is completely re-warmed, bypass is withdrawn, and the heart takes over the circulation again. The cannulas are then removed from the heart, the heparin reversed, haemostasis secured, and the chest closed.

Risk of perioperative death

The United Kingdom Cardiac Surgery Register provides an annual audit of mortality (in-hospital or 30 day) for all units, and is therefore the closest we have to a true average risk for all patients and all hospitals. This is of more interest to referring physicians than ideal figures from carefully selected series. During the early 1980s the falling death rate for coronary surgery levelled out and has remained remarkably consistent at between 2.5% and 2.7%.

The typical patient is a man less than 70 years old who has an elective operation for chronic stable angina. He will have three to four grafts, including a left internal mammary artery graft to the left anterior descending coronary artery. Some of the factors known to increase the risk of operative

61

death over and above those of this typical patient are summarised in the box above.

Perioperative morbidity after coronary surgery

Perioperative myocardial infarction

The incidence of perioperative myocardial infarction is debated, but if the usual criteria are used it may be as high as 10%. Discrete, anatomically localised, perioperative myocardial infarction characterised by new Q waves and loss of R waves is much less common, and clinically important acute regional myocardial damage is unusual. The incidence is influenced by surgical technique, in which case it results from occlusion of the grafted vessels or side branches of an artery in which an endarterectomy has been done. Methods of myocardial protection are designed to minimise myocardial ischaemia. More diffuse myocardial damage, indicated by leakage of enzymes and overall deterioration of left ventricular function, is more common but is less easy to define and the range of estimates of its incidence reflect this.

Low output state

Low output state, as a complication of operation, usually develops in patients who have poor preoperative left ventricular function, or those who come to theatre with an evolving infarction. Treatment should be supportive with intra-aortic balloon counterpulsation, reduction of afterload, and judicious use of inotropes. Some patients may be supported with mechanical assistance to the left ventricle in the hope that left ventricular function will recover. "Stunned myocardium" is well recognised and supportive treatment may result in excellent recovery once the heart is revascularised.

Arrhythmias after coronary surgery

The commonest arrhythmias after coronary surgery are atrial fibrillation and supraventricular tachycardia, which develop in 20–30% of all patients, usually about two to five days after operation. A wide range of prophylactic regimens have been suggested to reduce the incidence, including digoxin, calcium channel blockers, β-blockers, magnesium, and the maintenance of relative hyperkalaemia, but the incidence is essentially unchanged. The only important aetiological factors seem to be age and obesity, and perhaps hypoxia and left atrial distension are the intermediate mechanisms. Treatment is equally diverse, but fortunately the complication is (almost without exception) benign, controllable, and limited to the perioperative period. Acute ventricular arrhythmias, including fibrillation, are relatively uncommon but usually indicate perioperative ischaemia.

Morbidity after coronary artery surgery

Common and relatively benign
- Chest wall pain
- "Palpitations"
- Atrial arrhythmias
- Fluid retention and peripheral oedema
- Pleural effusions
- Low grade pyrexias
- Leg wound pain and inflammation

Rare but relatively important
- Sternal dehiscence
- Ventricular arrhythmias
- Heart block
- Pulmonary oedema and acute lung injury
- Deep vein thrombosis
- Pulmonary embolus

Heart block develops immediately after operation in a small proportion of patients, occasionally indicating an acute ischaemic event but more commonly as a temporary reaction to cardioplegic arrest. Persisting conduction abnormalities requiring permanent pacing are rare after coronary artery surgery.

Outlook after coronary surgery

The probability of a patient being alive a year after operation is 95%. Survival at five years is 88%, and remains good at 10 years when three quarters can expect to be alive. At least half of the deaths are caused by myocardial infarction or heart failure. There are some sudden deaths,

Outlook after coronary surgery	Percentage likelihood of being alive
At 30 days	97.5
At one year	95
At five years	88
At 10 years	75

presumably caused by heart block or ventricular fibrillation, as with native coronary artery disease.

Death, infarction, and the return of angina are more likely if revascularisation was incomplete, and their incidence correlates with subsequent graft occlusion. Progression of disease in the native system is a major contributory factor and it is probable that thorough attention to reducing risk factors will slow the rate of progression of both graft and native vessel disease. Secondary prevention with low dose aspirin improves the graft patency.

Recurrent angina

Early return of angina is probably caused by technical factors, either failure to bypass important stenoses or early occlusion of the anastomosis. Late recurrence of angina occurs with increasing frequency after five years. Assessment is the same as before the initial operation and the decision making process is similar. Many cases of mild angina can be managed medically. If operation is considered the decision making process is along the same lines as for a first operation but more weighted against surgery, because an estimate of the increased risk must be made, and the likelihood of technical success of a second operation is less.

Appendix: Anatomy of the coronary arteries

The coronary arteries arise as the first branches of the aorta. The left main coronary artery arises in the left sinus of Valsava, a dilatation in the root of the ascending aorta, and passes between the pulmonary artery and the left atrial appendage to reach the left atrioventricular groove. It is usually 1–2 cm long before it divides into the left anterior descending and left circumflex arteries.

The left anterior descending artery continues along the anterior interventricular sulcus to the apex of the heart and often passes round into the posterior interventricular sulcus. It provides branches to the right ventricular free wall, and larger branches to the left ventricular free wall and the interventricular septum. The left circumflex artery passes around the heart in the left atrioventricular groove for a variable distance, giving off branches, the obtuse marginal vessels that supply the lateral wall of the heart. If the coronary arterial circulation is left dominant, the circumflex rather than the right coronary artery gives rise to the posterior descending artery, in which case the branches supplying the posterolateral wall of the heart are called left posterolateral arteries. Variations in the anatomy of the circumflex artery are common.

The right coronary artery arises in the right sinus of Valsava and runs down the right atrioventricular groove to the crux of the heart where it makes a "U" turn and then terminates by bifurcating into the right posterior descending coronary artery and the right posterolateral coronary artery. The posterior descending coronary artery passes in the posterior interventricular groove for a variable length giving rise to septal, right, and left ventricular branches. It is common for the posterior descending coronary artery to arise before the crux, and its anatomy can be variable. The atrioventricular node artery arises at the apex of the "U" turn, and the sinus node artery often arises from the second or third centimetre of the right coronary artery.

6 Surgery for complications of ischaemic heart disease

- Evolving acute infarction or complications of angioplasty
- Mechanical complications of myocardial infarction
- Acute complications of myocardial infarction
- Chronic complications of ischaemic heart disease

Operation for evolving acute infarction or complications of angioplasty

It is unusual for a patient to be operated on acutely for an evolving acute infarction that occurred outside hospital. This is simply for logistic reasons, though there is little evidence of benefit from an operation undertaken under these circumstances. In the early days of coronary artery surgery it was attempted as it seemed to be the obvious way to try and save myocardium. Though some success was achieved, it became clear that the risks of the procedure were not outweighed by the benefits. We still do not know what is the best time to reopen an acutely occluded coronary artery, even with our present knowledge of thrombolysis, but it is unlikely that there is much to gain by reopening a vessel one or two hours after its occlusion, given the general risks of operating on a patient who has just had a myocardial infarction.

There are only two small groups of patients for whom emergency coronary artery surgery is indicated. Firstly, those who are already in hospital, and whose coronary anatomy is already known, may be helped by an emergency operation at the onset of symptoms. In practice, these are patients who are in

---

True emergency indications for coronary artery surgery

- Patients in hospital, with known coronary anatomy at the onset of symptoms
- After failed coronary angioplasty

---

a cardiac unit, and are awaiting coronary artery surgery. If an elective operation was justified for either symptomatic or prognostic reasons then it seems sensible to operate on these patients to interrupt and avert the course of their myocardial infarction. This happens only a few times a year even in a unit that does hundreds of coronary operations each year. The results are sufficiently good to justify this selective policy.

Secondly, there are a small number of patients who require emergency operations after coronary angioplasty. About 1–2% of all patients who undergo angioplasty will require emergency operations and in the United Kingdom this is about 150 cases a year.

Indications after failed angioplasty

Various events during or after coronary angioplasty may precipitate emergency operations, including increasing angina shortly after the angioplasty that does not respond to medical treatment and intractable ventricular fibrillation during the angioplasty. Patients who develop increasing angina after angioplasty usually have an acute occlusion of the artery that was treated. This can be the result of thrombosis at the site of the target lesion, local dissection of the coronary artery at the site of the target lesion, or dissection of the coronary artery itself caused by the intubation with the various catheters that are required for angioplasty.

Patients who are operated on for intractable ventricular fibrillation will die without operation, so for them there is no alternative. Patients who develop increasing angina after angioplasty are sometimes initially treated by repeat catheterisation and further angioplasty. Some of these patients require no further treatment, or they can be stabilised with devices such as intra-

---

Indications after failed angioplasty

- Intractable ventricular fibrillation during angioplasty
- Increasing angina after angioplasty
- Cardiogenic shock

---

coronary stents, but many will still need urgent operation to save their lives and preserve the myocardium, and considerations of long term prognosis are less important than after elective coronary operations.

The risk of dying after an emergency operation on the coronary arteries caused by failure of an angioplasty is undoubtedly increased over the risk of dying after elective coronary artery surgery, and this is particularly so for those who develop increasing angina during the hours after angioplasty. For a patient who is operated on having been transferred directly from the catheter laboratory in cardiogenic shock or ventricular fibrillation, the risks of the operation itself are irrelevant.

Controversy exists, however, about patients who are initially managed medically and whose symptoms deteriorate for some hours before they are transferred for emergency operation. It is clear that these patients are at an increased operative risk, though it is not clear exactly how great that risk is. It is also not clear whether the delay itself causes an increased risk over that that is incurred if the patient is operated on immediately after the failed angioplasty.

Operation

Cardiopulmonary bypass must be instituted rapidly. In a patient who has arrested either massage can be continued while the femoral vessels are exposed and cannulated, or massage can be interrupted briefly while the chest is draped and opened. One surgeon then embarks on internal massage while a second cannulates the femoral artery for cardiopulmonary bypass. Another strategy is to cannulate the aorta and right atrium, put the patient on bypass, and then to insert the purse strings to secure the bypass cannulas. The coronary artery surgery itself is done in the standard fashion. Only vein grafts should be used under these circumstances. An intra–aortic balloon pump may be inserted before attempts are made to wean the patient from cardiopulmonary bypass to try and reduce the requirements for inotropes and vasoconstricting agents.

There is some controversy about the use of the internal mammary artery for less seriously ill patients after failed angioplasty. We think that saphenous vein grafts should be used in preference to the internal mammary artery in unstable patients, as the objective is simply survival. In more stable patients using the internal mammary artery to graft the left anterior descending artery is not unreasonable, but it is sensible to insert a "back up" vein graft into a diagonal vessel.

Mechanical complications of myocardial infarction

If an area of heart muscle is deprived of its blood supply for more than about 20 minutes at 37°C, permanent damage with the death of myocytes begins. If the coronary artery obstruction is incomplete, the vessel reopens before all the myocytes have died, and if there is some perfusion from adjacent coronary arteries the infarction is patchy. If the obstruction is complete and unrelieved there is necrosis of the myocardium in that area and not only can it not contract, but it also has little tensile strength. The infarcted left ventricular muscle may rupture, which kills about 20% of patients who survive to reach hospital. Because it is a mechanical problem there is at least the possibility that these patients can be saved by operation if the diagnosis is made promptly, and if they survive long enough to have an operation. Only a few have a rupture that is amenable to repair and survive long enough to reach the operating theatre.

Acute complications of myocardial infarction

There are three typical patterns of acute myocardial rupture; rupture of the free wall of the ventricle, rupture of the interventricular septum and rupture of a papillary muscle.

Rupture of the free wall

This is the most common form of myocardial rupture and accounts for three quarters of the cases or about 15% of deaths in hospital in those who have survived for the first hours and days after myocardial infarction. It can occur at any time from the first few days to about three weeks after infarction.

The presentation is sudden deterioration of a patient apparently recovering from infarction. There is a loss of blood pressure and signs of cardiac tamponade. The rupture may be a full thickness rent with free communication between the ventricle and the pericardium, and survival is impossible. A few patients have been saved in whom the seepage of arterial blood has been contained by the epicardium or pericardial adhesions for long enough to have an emergency operation. Successful cases are unusual enough to feature as case reports. Cardiopulmonary bypass is instituted through cannulation of the femoral vessels before the chest is opened. The site of rupture is identified, the infarct is opened, and the free wall defect repaired with a Dacron cloth patch and Teflon buttressed sutures.

Patterns of acute myocardial rupture:

- Rupture of the free wall of the ventricle
- Rupture of the interventricular septum
- Rupture of a papillary muscle

69

Rupture of the ventricular septum

This is the second most common form of ventricular rupture. Estimates from necropsy figures suggest that it is the cause of death in only a few and it occurs in under 1% of all patients who have a diagnosis of myocardial infarction. There is characteristically a sudden deterioration between five days and a week after infarction. The patient has the typical signs of cardiogenic shock together with a precordial thrill and a pansystolic murmur. The differential diagnosis is ischaemic mitral regurgitation, and cross-sectional echo cardiography will differentiate between them. The usual management is operative repair if the patient has adequate remaining cardiac function. The mortality of operation is 25% to 50%, but, conservative management almost inevitably results in death.

Rupture of the ventricular septum occurs in one of two forms, anterior or posterior. They probably occur in roughly equal numbers, but anterior rupture of the interventricular septum is more common in surgical series as it has a slightly lower operative risk. The anterior rupture is usually associated with an acute occlusion of the left anterior descending coronary artery proximal to the origin of its first septal branch. It is common for the anterior descending coronary artery lesion to be the only major stenosis in the coronary artery tree, and for this reason there are few collaterals. The ensuing myocardial infarct tends to be extensive and full thickness, resulting in a "blow out" hole of the interventricular septum (fig 6.1). Occasionally one sees true ischaemic aneurysms of the interventricular septum, where the infarct has not ruptured, but has become thin and fibrous, exactly as in the more usual aneurysm of the free wall of the left ventricle. The posterior rupture of the interventricular septum is more likely to be associated with failure of the infarcted muscle to tolerate the local shear stresses at the junction of the septum and the right and left ventricles (see fig 6.2).

Areas of controversy in the management of rupture of the interventricular septum

The two main areas of controversy in the management of these patients are the timing of the operation, and whether or not to graft other diseased coronary vessels. The balance of opinion is towards early operation in those patients who have enough myocardial function remaining to survive. This includes the prophylactic insertion of an intra–aortic balloon pump before operation in those patients who are fit enough. Operation is the only treatment for these patients as all but a few will die if they do not have an operation. The problem lies in selecting those who have a reasonable chance of survival from those who will die whatever is done. Indicators of a worse prognosis are profound cardiogenic shock and the early onset of renal failure. Most reported series show that survival is worse if the rupture of the septum is posterior.

Controversy also exists whether or not to graft diseased coronary arteries in

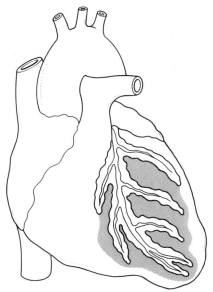

Figure 6.1 Site of rupture of an anterior post-infarction ventricular septal rupture (syn post-infarction ventricular septal defect).

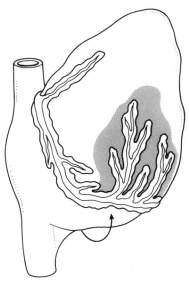

Figure 6.2 Site of rupture of a posterior post-infarction ventricular septal rupture (syn post-infarction ventricular septal defect).

71

non-infarcted territories of the heart. The overall results suggest that there is not additional risk associated with grafting, but there is also little evidence that it confers benefit. If one does not think that coronary artery grafting provides benefit in terms of survival there is no point in the delay and risk of doing coronary angiography in these patients. Certainly with the use of a Swan-Ganz catheter and high quality colour flow Doppler echocardiography there is no need to put the patients to the considerably increased risk of a left ventricular angiogram simply to confirm the diagnosis.

Prospects for survival

Without operation most patients will die within the first week, and many die within 24 hours of their presentation. Even with full supportive measures only a few survive to six weeks. Clearly the results of surgical management in this group of patients are skewed by the cases selected but overall about 60% of patients will survive repair of an anterior ventricular septal rupture. Most series report appreciably poorer survival after repair of posterior ventricular septal rupture. The use of blood cardioplegia and other developments in myocardial protection may improve these results.

Operation of repair of ventricular septal rupture

Cardiopulmonary bypass is instituted between superior and inferior vena caval drainage and ascending aortic return. Assuming that the coronary arteries are not going to be operated on, there are two alternatives: either the aorta can be cross-clamped and cardioplegia used for myocardial protection, or the heart can be fibrillated with the aorta left unclamped. Once the heart is widely open it cannot eject air and can therefore be defibrillated and allowed to beat. The ventricular septal rupture is identified after the heart has been opened through the area of the myocardial infarction. The defect is closed with a patch of Dacron cloth over the left ventricular side of the defect, and Teflon–felt buttressed sutures brought through from the right ventricular side of the defect (fig 6.3). With an anterior ventricular septal rupture it is usually possible to close the incision through the infarcted area simply by buttressing the incision with Teflon strips, but with a posterior ventricular septal rupture it is always necessary to place a patch at the site of ventriculotomy. The air is removed from the heart before it is finally closed, and after further removal of air the cross-clamp is released and the heart subsequently weaned from bypass. Most surgeons insert an intra-aortic balloon pump before attempting to wean the patient from bypass if one had not been inserted before operation.

Rupture of a papillary muscle

Rupture of a papillary muscle causes acute mitral regurgitation and the severity of the damage to the muscle governs the severity of the mitral

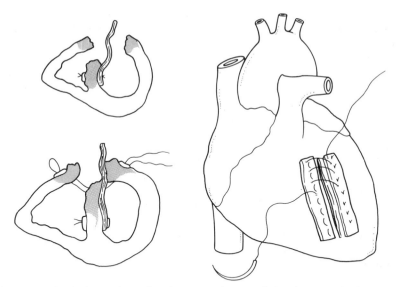

Figure 6.3 Technique of repair of an anterior post-infarction ventricular septal rupture.

regurgitation. Mild papillary muscle ischaemia will produce mild mitral regurgitation, and complete rupture of the papillary muscle will produce torrential mitral regurgitation and cardiogenic shock. Management depends on the severity of the mitral regurgitation, and surgical repair is done for severe mitral regurgitation in a patient who has adequate remaining cardiac function.

Operation for papillary muscle rupture

A standard mitral valve operation is done, but it can be technically more difficult than usual as the left atrium tends to be of normal size, rather than enlarged as in chronic mitral regurgitation. These patients are often so ill that they require support with inotropes or the insertion of an intra-aortic balloon pump, or both, before they are taken to the operating theatre. After median sternotomy, cardiopulmonary bypass is instituted between superior and inferior vena caval drainage and ascending aortic return, the ascending aorta is cross-clamped, and the heart is arrested with cardioplegia. The left atrium is opened and the mitral valve inspected. Any necessary distal coronary artery bypass grafts are then done, after which the mitral valve is repaired, or excised and replaced, as appropriate. After air has been removed the cross-clamp is released, and the heart reperfused. During rewarming the proximal vein graft anastomoses are completed, after which the patient can be weaned

73

from cardiopulmonary bypass. Because of the recent myocardial infarction, it is common for these patients to require support with either inotropes or an intra-aortic balloon pump for a period after their operation. Overall operative mortality is 10–20%, depending on the severity of myocardial damage and the need for procedures other than replacement of the mitral valve.

Chronic complications of ischaemic heart disease

Apart from chronic left ventricular failure, there are three major chronic complications of ischaemic heart disease. Chronic mitral regurgitation is a result of dilation of the mitral annulus, and its management will be considered in chapter 7. The formation of a left ventricular aneurysm and the development of ventricular arrhythmias in association with a subendocardial scar are the other two problems.

Left ventricular aneurysms

Formation of a left ventricular aneurysm results from a full thickness regional myocardial infarct (fig 6.4). Characteristically this occurs in the territory of the left anterior descending artery, usually when the artery has been obstructed proximal to its first diagonal branch. Once the myocytes have died, the scar thins and the fibres slip, so that the total number of muscle fibres in the wall of the scar is reduced. In the classical description of a ventricular aneurysm, the aneurysmal segment will expand in ventricular systole, and contract by recoil in ventricular diastole. Sometimes this can clearly be seen on the angiogram. The presence of clot within the cavity of the aneurysm (which is common), may reduce its apparent size at angiography. In these circumstances, echocardiography can help in the assessment of these patients.

Operation is undertaken for one of three reasons: to reduce the chances of embolisation of mural thrombus from the inner surface of the aneurysm, to prevent recurrent episodes of ventricular tachycardia or fibrillation, and to reduce the rate of deterioration into severe chronic heart failure. Operating to reduce the risk of systemic embolisation of mural thrombus alone is a "soft" indication unless the patient has had systemic signs of embolisation; usually one will prescribe warfarin and ensure regular echocardiographic follow-up. Operation for ventricular arrhythmias is discussed later in this chapter. Operation for heart failure is unpredictable: in a patient with a large well–defined aneurysm and obvious symptoms it can be rewarding, and there is evidence that newer, more sophisticated, forms of ventricular repair can produce good functional benefit. In patients with less well-defined aneurysms the mechanical (and therefore the symptomatic) benefit is less. In patients

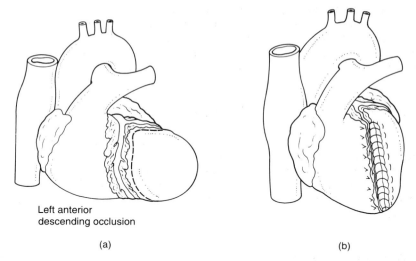

Left anterior
descending occlusion

(a)   (b)

Figure 6.4 The development of a left ventricular aneurysm, and a technique of repair.

such as these an operation might be done as part of a coronary artery procedure when it might not be indicated on its own.

Overall the operative mortality is about 4% for isolated repair of a left ventricular aneurysm, and about 8% when combined with coronary artery bypass grafting.

Operation for left ventricular aneurysm

Cardiopulmonary bypass is instituted between superior and inferior vena caval drainage and ascending aortic return. Assuming that the coronary arteries are not going to be operated on, there are two alternatives: either the aorta can be cross-clamped and cardioplegia used for myocardial protection,

---

Left ventricular aneurysms

Indications for operation:
- Reduce the risk of systemic embolisation
- Prevent ventricular arrhythmias
- To treat heart failure

Operative risk:
- 4% to 8%

---

or the heart can be fibrillated with the aorta left unclamped. Once the heart is widely open it can be defibrillated and allowed to beat. In the classic technique of linear suture, the aneurysm is trimmed back to a rim of strong fibrous tissue next to viable myocardium, and the defect repaired by direct suture of the two edges of fibrous scar. This generally does not require buttressing with Teflon-felt strips as the fibrous tissue holds stitches well; this is in contrast to the repair of a ventriculotomy after acute ventricular septal rupture. The technique of linear suture results in distortion of the cavity of the left ventricle, and more recent techniques have been introduced to attempt to return the geometry of the left ventricle to a more normal shape, to redistribute wall stress in a more physiological fashion, and to improve ventricular performance. Having closed the heart, air is removed and the cross-clamp released. After rewarming has been completed the patient is weaned from bypass.

Ventricular tachyarrhythmias and subendocardial scars

Only a few patients with ischaemic heart disease develop sustained ventricular tachycardia, but when they do it is usually in association with a left ventricular aneurysm. As a group, patients with sustained ventricular tachycardia and ischaemic heart disease have worse left ventricular function than those with ischaemic heart disease alone. The focus of sustained ventricular tachycardia is related to a subendocardial scar in which there is a mixture of viable myocardial tissue and fibrous scarring. Preoperative electrophysiological mapping is important to identify the site of the focus, as occasionally electrophysiological mapping at operation does not induce the tachycardia or localise the site of the focus. We are looking for the area of earliest endocardial activation that precedes the QRS complex during sustained ventricular tachycardia. This will precede the QRS complex by between 20 and 80 milliseconds and often lies on the ventricular septum near the border of an aneurysm or infarct.

Operation is recommended for those patients who have life threatening arrhythmias confirmed by electrophysiological testing while they are taking appropriate antiarrhythmic drugs. Not surprisingly because of the poor left ventricular function in this group of patients, operative mortality is relatively high. Cardiogenic shock is the most common mode of death in the early perioperative period. Longer term survival is similarly limited by the degree of heart failure, and the survival curves are similar to those seen in patients with moderate to severe heart failure. Overall only half these patients will be alive five years after their operation, and most die within three months of operation.

Operation for ventricular tachycardia

Cardiopulmonary bypass is instituted between superior and inferior vena caval drainage and ascending aortic return. The heart may be fibrillated with the aorta left unclamped. Once the heart is widely open it can be defibrillated and allowed to beat. The ventricle is opened through the area of infarction or aneurysm and the focus of the tachycardia identified by electrophysiological mapping. The area of subendocardium is then excised and the resection margin is ablated after which the electrophysiological mapping is repeated. If the focus has been ablated, the heart is closed and air removed before the patient is weaned from bypass. Patches for an automatic internal converting defibrillator may be applied to the heart at this time if appropriate, though now it is more common to insert such systems as a whole transvenously if and when they are indicated. Additional operations for coronary artery disease can be done at the same time if indicated.

7 Surgery for valvar heart disease

- Repair or replacement in valve surgery
- Choice of artificial heart valve
- Pathological changes, indications for operation, and operative techniques for the individual valves
- Endocarditis
- Postoperative management of valvar heart disease
- Appendix: anatomy of the cardiac valves

Valve disease is essentially mechanical and therefore particularly amenable to surgical correction. Function can be restored by valve repair, or more frequently, the valve may be replaced. Lesions of the valves endanger life in a number of ways. There may be gradually worsening cardiac damage and disability (which is a feature of chronic mitral stenosis), severe acute heart failure (as in acute mitral or aortic regurgitation), or sudden death may result from severe aortic stenosis.

The indications for and timing of operation require careful thought, with a clear appreciation of the risks and benefits in each individual patient. The risks and benefits of the procedures vary, so it is necessary to know about not only the underlying pathological processes and their history under medical treatment, but also about the problems associated with the operation itself, be it repair or replacement. A replacement valve has inherent risks, including the need for lifelong anticoagulation for mechanical valves, the risks of valve failure and thromboembolism, and the continuing risk of endocarditis. Even after successful valve replacement there is an annual valve–related mortality of 1–2% and this must be borne in mind together with the natural history of the valve lesion itself, when deciding on the appropriate time for operation.

After the initial decision to operate on a valve, there are two further decisions that must be made. Firstly do you expect that the valve will be repairable? Secondly, if the valve is to be replaced what prosthesis should be selected?

Repair or replacement in valve surgery

Because there are always risks associated with prosthetic valves, interest has continued in methods to repair the native valves. The argument for repair or replacement turns on the long term outcome of the two procedures, and the timing of the operation. If repair is possible, then preservation of the native valve should provide the patient with the best available valve. In other words an abnormal but functioning native valve is better than any current prosthetic valve. In practical terms, however, repair is an option only in the mitral and tricuspid valves. Repair often takes longer than replacement and has a less sure haemodynamic outcome; in particular there is an increased risk of regurgitation through a repaired valve. For this reason there is a wide difference of opinion about the indications for repair as opposed to replacement. Enthusiasts repair quite severely damaged valves, whereas others will replace valves that are relatively normal in anatomical but not functional terms.

Repair of the aortic valve

In adult practice it is unusual to repair an aortic valve if the aortic root itself is not diseased. Commissurotomy in aortic stenosis is possible, but it is generally reserved for congenital aortic stenosis in infants and small children. Commissurotomy in adult calcific or rheumatic aortic stenosis almost invariably results in uncontrollable aortic regurgitation, together with maintenance of an appreciable gradient across the valve because the cusps remain too stiff to open and close normally. This is directly analogous to our experience with percutaneous balloon dilatation of the aortic valve in elderly patients, long term results of which are poor. Ultrasonic decalcification has been attempted during open operations to overcome the stiffness of the valve leaflets, but this has not resulted in long term success.

Repair of the aortic valve is often undertaken in patients who have an acute dissection of the ascending aorta with prolapse of the aortic valve caused by disruption of the commissural attachments of the leaflet tissue. Under these circumstances it is generally possible to reconstitute the commissural attachments to the aortic wall before repair of the aortic dissection. In many ways this is better thought of as repair of the supporting structure of the valve rather than repair of the valve itself. Repair and replacement of aortic leaflets with autologous pericardium treated with glutaraldehyde has also been described, but this procedure is undertaken in only a few centres, and results of long term follow up are awaited.

Repair of the mitral valve

In contrast to the aortic valve, there is considerable experience in repairing the mitral valve. Mitral stenosis was the first of the valve lesions to be amenable to surgical correction, and the technique of closed mitral valvotomy was first undertaken in 1948. This has largely been superseded by open mitral valvotomy or balloon mitral valvotomy in western countries, but it is still widely used in regions of the world where rheumatic fever is common. In the United Kingdom only eleven closed mitral valvotomies were done during 1990, whereas many units in the Asian subcontinent will do two or three such procedures a day. Balloon mitral valvotomy has the same effect as closed mitral valvotomy, but uses a balloon under radiographic control to open up the fused commissures of the stenotic mitral valve rather than a dilator under digital control.

Mitral valve surgery has become more sophisticated since the advent of cardiopulmonary bypass and there are a number of issues to consider in surgery of the mitral valve. These include the state of the mitral annulus, the nature of the tissues of the leaflets, and the state of the subvalvar apparatus. If the main abnormality is mitral stenosis with fusion of the commissures these can be divided as can the underlying chordae tendineae. When this is done as an open operation it is analogous to the classic closed mitral valvotomy for rheumatic mitral stenosis or the current percutaneous balloon dilatation of the mitral valve. If the haemodynamic lesion is mitral regurgitation, the anatomy of the valve will dictate which procedure is done.

Decision making in valvar heart disease

- Which valve?
  Aortic, mitral, tricuspid or a combination
- Disease
  Regurgitation, stenosis or both
- Potential for repair
  Never in aortic, possible in mitral, usual in tricuspid
- Choice of prosthetic valve
  Pre-existing need for long term anticoagulation
  Mechanical, xenograft, homograft
- Associated coronary artery disease or other cardiac conditions
- Special cases – for example, child-bearing women
- Timing of operation

Indications for mitral valve surgery:

- Mitral stenosis
- Annular dilatation
- Excessive leaflet tissue,
- Prolapse of leaflets

If the main abnormality is annular dilatation, the annulus can be narrowed with a prosthetic ring which is implanted to support it. Part of the posterior leaflet may be resected to prevent the development of redundant leaflet tissue after the annulus has been reduced in diameter.

If the primary problem is excessive leaflet tissue, there are instances where it is possible to produce a competent valve merely by resecting the excess leaflet tissue, but under these circumstances the annulus is usually repaired at the same time (see fig 7.1).

If the main abnormality is prolapse of the leaflet caused by rupture or elongation of the chordae, the damaged chordae may be repaired or replaced. Alternatively the appropriate region of the leaflet may be resected and replaced by transferring another chorda into that part of the leaflet. An annuloplasty will usually be done at the same time.

Repair of the tricuspid valve

In adults operation on the tricuspid valve is much less common than operation on the mitral valve. Tricuspid stenosis is rare and almost invariably results from rheumatic fever, and tricuspid incompetence can be caused by rheumatic fever or is simply an indication of right ventricular overload. Like mitral stenosis, tricuspid stenosis can be treated by commissurotomy, but tricuspid incompetence requires either annuloplasty or occasionally replacement.

Repair of the pulmonary valve

In adults operation on the pulmonary valve is unusual; occasionally pulmonary valvotomy may be done for late presentation of congenital pulmonary stenosis.

Choice of artificial heart valve

Types of valves

If you have decided to implant an artificial valve into a patient you have also to decide which valve you will use. There are three groups available:

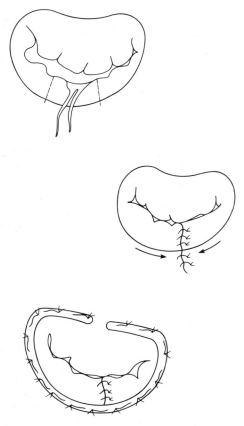

Figure 7.1 Repair of the mitral valve, showing a quadrangular resection of the centre of the posterior leaflet, repair of the defect, and the insertion of an annuloplasty ring.

firstly, the mechanical valves which are made from materials such as Silastic, pyrolytic carbon, and titanium steel. Secondly, there are xenograft valves, which are prepared from biological tissue such as porcine aortic valves or sheets of bovine pericardium and then mounted in an artificial frame called a "stent". These are often called "tissue valves". Thirdly, there are homografts, which are human valves that are recovered from cadavers or explanted hearts at transplantation; they are not mounted in a stent. There is a fourth group that has recently been introduced, which are stentless xenograft valves and these are used in a similar way to homografts.

Mechanical valves

There are three groups of mechanical valves. The first are the "ball in

82

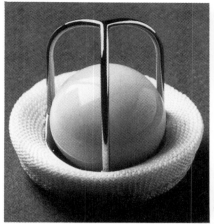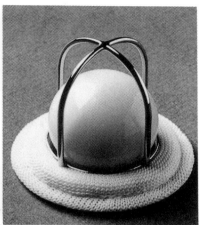

Figure 7.2 (a) A "ball in cage" aortic prosthetic heart valve (note the three struts). (b) A "ball in cage" mitral prosthetic heart valve (note the four struts). (Photograph courtesy of Baxter.)

cage" valves, in which a Silastic ball moves to and fro within a metal cage with three struts for an aortic valve and four struts for a mitral valve (figs 7.2a and 7.2b). When blood flows through the valve the ball moves away from the seating as far as it can within the cage, and when the valve is closed the ball is seated in the ring of the cage.

The second group are the monoleaflet valves. A circular disc moves from its closed position where the occluding disc is lying on the seating ring, to an open position where the disc is at an angle to the seating ring. In this type of valve much of the blood flow through the valve is through its centre.

In the third group, the bileaflet valves, there are two semi-circular leaflets each of which rotates through 90° from a closed position to an open position. In these valves most of the blood flow is through the central orifice of the valve (see fig 7.3).

Xenograft valves

There are two main groups of xenograft valves. The first are aortic valves from pigs which are selected, fixed in glutaraldehyde, and then inserted into prosthetic frames called "stents". The function of the stent is to give mechanical support to the valve to maintain its competence, and to provide a convenient way in which the valve can be sewn into the appropriate position in the heart. These valves vary among different manufacturers in the exact method of fixation and the design of the mounting stent (see fig 7.4).

The second type of xenograft valves are made from sheets of bovine pericardium which are cut to the appropriate shape and then mounted on a

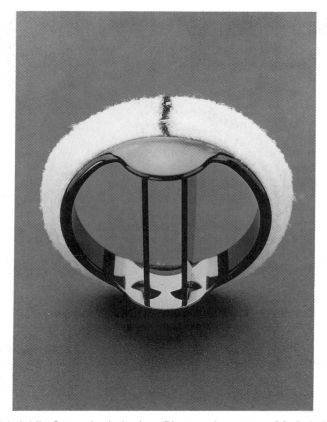

Figure 7.3 A bileaflet mechanical valve. (Photograph courtesy of St Jude Medical.)

frame, again called a stent, which mimics the shape of a natural aortic valve. Again the pericardium is fixed in glutaraldehyde and the valves vary among manufacturers, there being variations in the method of fixation, the design of the mounting stent, and the way in which the pericardium is sewn to it.

Homograft valves

Homograft valves are excised from human hearts. They are stored in various ways, including tissue culture medium, antibiotic solution, and liquid nitrogen. Both pulmonary and aortic valves can be used for homograft valves, and, for example, a complete aortic root may be used. The availability of homografts is obviously relatively limited as both the heart itself and the donor from which it came have to be suitable. In particular the valves must be anatomically normal and mechanically in good condition, and the donor must be free of potentially transferable illness.

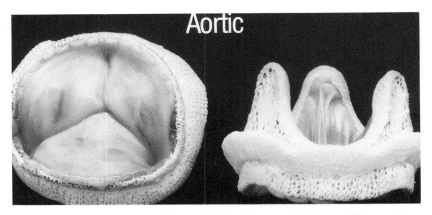

Figure 7.4 A porcine xenograft (tissue) valve. (Photograph courtesy of Baxter.)

Recently porcine valves have been prepared in a similar way to homografts, with a view to providing the benefits of homografts together with wider availability, and in particular a wider choice of sizes (see fig 7.5).

The choice of valve

The choice of valve must be tailored to the individual patient, particularly as each type of replacement valve has both advantages and disadvantages. Patients given any of the mechanical valves currently available will have to take anticoagulants, usually warfarin, for the rest of their lives. Balanced against this though is that one can expect any implanted mechanical valve to last for the duration of the patient's life. There are now recorded examples of early types of mechanical valve that have lasted for over 30 years, and at around 45 million heart beats/year or 1.35 billion heart beats in total, this is most impressive.

The xenograft valves do not need anticoagulating for life, but some mitral valves are anticoagulated for a short time in the early postoperative period.

Valves:

- Mechanical – require anticoagulation for life, but last
- Xenograft – do not require anticoagulation, but wear out
- Homografts – availability limited and difficult to insert, but good haemodynamic characteristics and last longer than xenografts

---

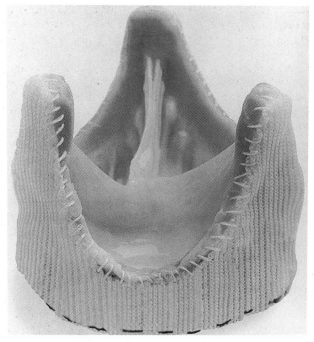

Figure 7.5 A stentless porcine xenograft valve. (Photograph courtesy of St Jude Medical.)

Xenografts undergo mechanical wear, however, and will inevitably fail at some point, usually but not always, slowly and with adequate warning.

The homografts share many of the problems of the xenografts, availability is limited and they are more difficult to insert. They do, however, have good haemodynamic characteristics and probably last longer than xenografts.

The minimal risk of failure of mechanical valves might suggest that they would be used in all cases, but any patient with a mechanical valve must be anticoagulated permanently to reduce if not prevent the risk of thromboembolism arising from the valve, or thrombosis of the valve itself. Taking warfarin has its own risks, in particular it is difficult to control the dose, and the risks of thromboembolism and bleeding tend to negate the benefit of potentially limitless durability.

In older patients, in whom it could be reasonably expected that the xenograft valve would last 10 to 15 years and that this would be adequate to exceed the patient's life expectancy it may be that either the valves fail earlier than expected, or that the patients survive longer than expected. This presents the problem of the elderly patient in whom reoperation on the valve may be necessary, at both increased risk to the patient and further cost. As a result of this the lower age limit for inserting a xenograft valve has gradually increased, and most centres now reserve them for patients over the age of 70 years.

There are, of course, exceptions to this rule – for example, young women who wish to have families, for whom warfarin is contraindicated because of its teratogenicity. The problem is further compounded as xenografts tend to fail more quickly in younger patients, and though a homograft would be an acceptable compromise for an aortic valve, it would not be appropriate for a mitral valve. One approach would be to attempt to repair the mitral valve, and if this fails a xenograft should be used. The patient must be aware that it will require replacement in a relatively short time, and that the risks of reoperation will be slightly more than those of the initial operation. Alternatively if a mechanical valve is inserted, the conventional teaching is that the patient should be given heparin rather than warfarin before conception and this should be continued for the first trimester. Warfarin should then be given for the second trimester and heparin for the final trimester.

Choosing between the types of mechanical or xenograft valves is often difficult. The bileaflet mechanical valves have better haemodynamic behaviour than the ball–in–cage type, but the ball–in–cage type have been followed up for longer and are usually cheaper. Between the xenograft valves, the pericardial valves particularly the smaller sizes, are often claimed to have a better haemodynamic profile, but the stented porcine xenografts seem to be more durable. The true homografts last longer than the xenograft analogues whereas the xenograft analogues are available in a wider range of sizes "off the shelf" and are a little easier to insert.

Pathological changes, indications for operation, and operative techniques for the individual valves

The timing of operation on any particular valve lesion or combination of lesions depends on judgement of the point at which the risks of the natural history of the disease outweigh the risks of the operation itself and the risks associated with an implanted prosthetic valve. This in turn depends on an understanding of both the natural history of the disease, the effects of medical management on the natural history, and the operative risks for any particular patient. As previously discussed, it also requires an understanding of the risks of a prosthetic valve, including the incidence of thromboembolism and anticoagulant–related haemorrhage.

To simplify the discussion of the surgical techniques of valve replacement we will assume that the technique of cold antegrade crystalloid cardioplegia is used throughout.

Signs and symptoms of aortic stenosis

- Angina
- Ejection systolic murmur
- Slow rising pulse
- Breathlessness on exertion
- Malaise, tiredness

Aortic stenosis

The aortic valve usually presents no resistance to flow, the peak systolic aortic pressure being the same as the peak ventricular systolic pressure. Blood flow is usually obstructed at the valve, although it may occasionally be caused by lesions above or below the valve. Classic adult aortic stenosis results from one of three diseases: rheumatic fever with commissural fusion, leaflet thickening, and subsequent calcification, as in the mitral valve. Secondly, a degenerative process can occur in a congenitally bicuspid valve as it thickens and calcifies; this is more common than severe congenital stenosis presenting in neonates or infants. Thirdly, it is becoming increasingly common to see degenerative processes with leaflet and annular calcification in tricuspid aortic valves in elderly patients. As the population ages and rheumatic fever becomes increasingly rare, the proportion of patients with the third pattern of disease will increase.

As the obstruction becomes more severe the ventricle has to generate excess pressure to overcome the obstruction and maintain the systolic pressure in the aorta. This results in hypertrophy of the left ventricular myocardium with an increasing demand for oxygen by the myocardium. As the disease progresses the frequency of ventricular arrhythmias increases.

Symptoms, signs, and investigations in aortic stenosis

There are three characteristic presenting symptoms, and once they have appeared the median survival without valve replacement is under two years. Angina, indistinguishable from that of coronary artery disease may occur. In this age group coronary artery disease may coexist, but the presence of an ejection systolic murmur and a slow rising pulse will indicate the presence of an important degree of aortic stenosis. Effort syncope, is a dramatic presentation which can be fatal. External cardiac massage of these patients can be difficult as they tend to have hypertrophied, stiff hearts with normal end diastolic volumes. Breathlessness on exertion, malaise, and general weariness are common. Unfortunately the signs often develop slowly and are so non-specific that the underlying aortic valve disease may be unrecognised.

The classic signs are a slow rising pulse, a forceful apex beat, and an ejection systolic murmur radiating to the carotids (fig 7.6). The ECG shows electrical left ventricular hypertrophy and there may be poststenotic dilation of the ascending aorta in the chest x ray film. Only late in the disease is the left ventricle obviously enlarged. Echocardiography with Doppler measurements of the gradient is the initial investigation, and will usually be followed by left heart catheterisation, left ventriculography, and coronary angiography.

Indications for aortic valve replacement in aortic stenosis

Aortic valve replacement is indicated for patients with symptomatic aortic stenosis, and the degree of urgency is increased if there is evidence of heart failure and angina. Patients with a gradient above 60 mmHg should be offered an operation on prognostic grounds, even in the absence of symptoms. Gradients above 80 mmHg are usually considered to be an indication for an operation "soon" and gradients above 100 mmHg for "urgent" operation. Syncopal episodes are an indication for a "very urgent" operation.

Aortic regurgitation

Aortic regurgitation results from either disease of the aortic annulus, or from disease of the leaflets themselves. Dilatation of the aortic annulus may be caused by a number of processes including systemic hypertension, connective tissue disease such as Marfan's syndrome, aneurysmal dilatation of the aorta in association with atherosclerosis, and acute dissection of the aortic wall. Diseases of the leaflets include rheumatic fever, connective tissue disease, and infective endocarditis. Mild to moderate aortic regurgitation can be present with minimal symptoms and has a reasonably stable course over time. The commoner symptoms include breathlessness, particularly on exercise, palpitations, and (occasionally) non-specific chest pain.

Indications for operation in aortic regurgitation

Indications for operation include worsening symptoms and evidence that the ventricle is starting to dilate. The most useful indices are enlargement of the heart in the x ray film to greater than half the cardiothoracic ratio, or evidence on echocardiography that the end-systolic dimension has increased to over 55 mm. Severe aortic regurgitation should be treated at presentation to prevent ventricular damage, even if it is relatively asymptomatic. The sudden onset of aortic regurgitation is poorly tolerated and requires urgent operation.

Surgery of the aortic valve

Aortic valves are repaired only rarely, unless the patient has an aortic dissection, and they are almost invariably replaced. The chest is opened through a standard median sternotomy and the heart is exposed. The

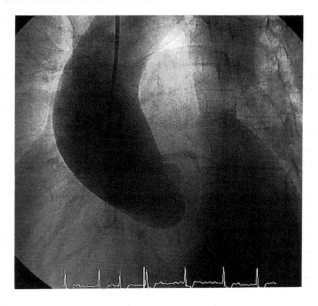

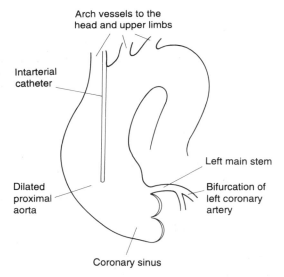

Figure 7.6 Aortogram by intra-arterial injection of contrast into the ascending aorta showing the sinuses of Valsalva (the coronary sinuses) and a dilated ascending aorta in association with aortic stenosis.

ascending aorta is cannulated, the exact site varying according to the surgeon's preference and the presence of palpable plaques in the wall of the aorta, but the cannula is placed to allow space to place an aortic cross–clamp and to open the aorta. In practice, this usually means that the aorta is cannulated distal to the pericardial reflection. The right atrium is cannulated with a single venous cannula and bypass begun. The patient is cooled, the ascending aorta is cross–clamped, and one litre of ice cold cardioplegia is given. When electromechanical arrest has been achieved the ascending aorta is opened and the aortic valve exposed. In severe aortic regurgitation it may be necessary to open the ascending aorta and give the cardioplegia directly into the orifices of the coronary arteries to prevent the heart distending.

The aortic valve is then excised and the aortic annulus decalcified; great care is taken to aspirate any loose debris, and the valve is then sized and the appropriate replacement selected. The replacement valve is sewn into place, and a further bolus of cardioplegia is given as about 30 minutes will have elapsed. Finally the aorta is closed as the patient is rewarmed. Air is removed from the aorta and the heart; the aortic cross-clamp is released, and the heart allowed to reperfuse. If sinus rhythm does not return spontaneously, defibrillation, or pacing, or both are undertaken until a satisfactory cardiac action is achieved. After the patient has been weaned from bypass the atrial cannula is removed and the heparin reversed with protamine. Any blood remaining in the cardiopulmonary bypass circuit is transfused, and then the aortic cannula is removed. Generally a single right ventricular pacing wire is placed before the chest is closed as the occasional patient will develop heart block in the early perioperative period.

The operative mortality in the United Kingdom for isolated aortic replacement in 1990 was 4.1% for mechanical prostheses, 4.7% for xenograft replacements, and 7.1% for homograft replacements. These figures do not differentiate between operations for aortic stenosis and aortic regurgitation.

Mitral stenosis

Mitral stenosis is a consequence of acute rheumatic fever in childhood or adolescence, the valve disease varying from mild commissural fusion with a pliable valve and relatively normal chordae (fig 7.7a), to severe commissural fusion with associated chordal shortening and fusion (fig 7.7b). There will be associated calcification of the leaflets confined to the valve leaflets in the milder forms, but extending through the annulus into the wall of the ventricle in the severest forms (fig 7.7c). In severe disease the valve orifice can be reduced from a normal size of about 2 by 3 cm to a tiny orifice of less than 1 by 0.5 cm. The normal valve orifice is 4–8 cm^2, but most patients coming to operation have valve orifices of less than 1.5 cm^2.

Symptoms, signs and investigation of mitral stenosis

The characteristic symptoms of mitral stenosis are breathlessness, both on

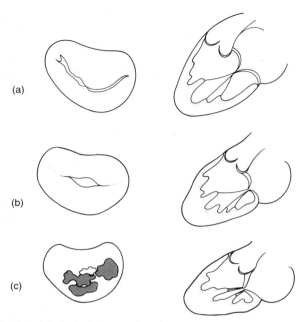

(a)

(b)

(c)

Figure 7.7 The pathological changes in mitral stenosis.

exertion and lying flat, together with palpitations, fatigue, and general malaise. The stenotic valve obstructs blood flow from the left atrium to the left ventricle, and the symptoms are caused by raised left atrial pressure and reduced cardiac output. The raised left atrial pressure results in raising of the pulmonary venous, and therefore pulmonary capillary, pressure. If this comes close to or exceeds the plasma oncotic pressure (which is normally about 25 mmHg) the alveoli and pulmonary interstitium become loaded with fluid. This impairs oxygenation, changes lung compliance, and causes breathlessness. This sensation is exacerbated by any manoeuvre that increases venous return, and further increases the pulmonary capillary pressure. Exercise (which increases blood flow) and lying down (which encourages the return of blood to the heart) both commonly precipitate episodes of acute breathlessness.

In some patients the back pressure results in a series of progressive changes in the right heart. These include pulmonary arterial hypertension, right ventricular dilatation, right ventricular failure, and tricuspid regurgitation. These can lead to all the signs of raised right atrial pressure including peripheral oedema, hepatic enlargement and engorgement, and both pleural effusions and ascites.

The characteristic signs of mitral stenosis include a tapping apex beat and a number of ausculatory findings. There is a loud first sound as the valve which has been held open for much longer than normal abruptly closes as ventricular pressure rises. There is a loud opening snap as the high left atrial pressure abruptly opens the valve at the beginning of diastole, and the low pitched diastolic flow murmur, which is most prominent at the apex with the patient turned slightly to the left.

The single most useful investigation in mitral stenosis remains the echocardiogram which is non-invasive, relatively simple, and cheap. With increasing use of transoesophageal echocardiography this investigation is becoming more invasive and probably slightly less safe, but the reward is better visualisation of the valve and the flow patterns through the valve. On echocardiography the valve can be seen moving, its thickness and mobility assessed, and the extent to which it is stenotic or regurgitant judged. Many patients are of an age at which silent coronary artery disease is common, and at least for this reason they will require cardiac catheterisation to measure both left and right heart pressures, as well as a left ventriculogram and coronary angiogram.

Timing of operation

The timing of operation depends on symptoms, the degree of mitral stenosis, and the nature of the valve. As in all aspects of medicine, the general rules of treating to relieve symptoms, to improve prognosis, or as a combination of both, apply. If low risks together with high rewards are possible then early operation is essential. For example, a patient with severe symptoms and an irreparable valve needs an urgent operation. A patient who has only moderate symptoms and an irreparable valve might be followed up closely, whereas another patient with similar symptoms and a valve suitable for a valvotomy rather than replacement would be considered for an early operation. This would be on the grounds that appreciable benefit could be achieved with both a low operative risk and a low risk of needing a replacement valve. A history of severe acute decompensation during pregnancy, systemic embolisation, or an atrial thrombus, are all indications for urgent operation. A patient who is breathless on moderate exercise, lying flat, or episodically at night, has got severe symptoms.

Signs and symptoms of mitral stenosis

- Acute breathlessness both on exertion and at rest
- Palpitations
- Peripheral oedema
- Enlargement and engorgement of liver
- Pleural effusion, ascites

Mitral regurgitation

The aetiology of mitral regurgitation is reflected in the anatomy of the valve. Mitral regurgitation can occur as a result of disease of the annulus, of the leaflet tissue, or of the tensioning apparatus. Annular dilatation can occur in an anatomically normal valve as a consequence of left ventricular dilatation, or of disease of the annulus itself. Excess valve tissue can prolapse into the left atrium, or the valve tissue can be perforated by endocarditis. Alternatively, the leaflets can contract and fail to oppose. The chordae tendineae may elongate or rupture, and the papillary muscles may cease to function, or even rupture as a consequence of ischaemic heart disease and myocardial infarction.

Symptoms, signs and investigation of mitral regurgitation

The mechanism of mitral regurgitation is similar to that of mitral stenosis, with raised left atrial pressure being transmitted back to the pulmonary capillaries. The severity of symptoms depends on both the volume of regurgitant blood and the size and compliance of the left atrium. A large and compliant left atrium can handle a far larger degree of mitral regurgitation before symptoms develop than a small and non-compliant left atrium. The most common symptom is shortness of breath, and like mitral stenosis this is exacerbated by exercise or lying down.

The chest radiograph will show an enlarged left atrium, and echocardiography—particularly with colour flow mapping—is diagnostic. Cardiac catheterisation with right and left heart pressure tracings, left ventriculography, and coronary angiography should be done before operation.

Timing of operation for mitral regurgitation

The timing of operation depends on the patient's general condition, whether the mitral regurgitation is acute or chronic, and whether it is secondary to another treatable process, the treatment of which could be expected to allow the mitral regurgitation to reverse.

Most patients who present with sudden acute severe mitral regurgitation rapidly develop pulmonary oedema and require urgent operation. A few stabilise on intensive medical treatment with vasodilators and diuretics and can be operated on electively. Patients who present with severe symptoms will require operation in the near future, while patients with more moderate symptoms can be assessed on the degree of mitral regurgitation and their left ventricular function. Patients who have signs of deteriorating left ventricular function should be operated on, while those whose left ventricular function is good can be followed up by chest radiography and echocardiography at regular intervals.

Patients with combined mild to moderate mitral regurgitation and left ventricular dysfunction together with coronary artery disease may present a diagnostic conundrum. Some will benefit from mitral valve replacement at the time of their coronary surgery; others will not need mitral valve replacement; and a third group will need early reoperation for mitral valve replacement that was not done at the time of their coronary artery surgery. Increasing experience with mitral valve repair is leading some surgeons to explore and repair the mitral valve at the time of coronary artery surgery when it would previously have been left untouched.

Surgery of the mitral valve

The chest is opened through a standard median sternotomy and the heart exposed. Heparin is given and the heart cannulated for cardiopulmonary bypass. The ascending aorta is cannulated to allow space to place an aortic cross–clamp and a cardioplegia cannula. The right atrium is cannulated with two venous cannulas, one through the atrial appendage and into the superior vena cava, and the other through a separate atrial purse string and into the inferior vena cava. Bypass is then started, the patient is cooled, the ascending aorta is cross–clamped, and one litre of ice cold cardioplegia is given. After electromechanical arrest the left atrium is opened and the mitral valve exposed. There are a number of different approaches to the mitral valve, the commonest being an incision in the left atrium that starts below the right superior pulmonary vein and passes posteriorly behind the inferior vena cava in the free wall of the left atrium.

The mitral valve is exposed and inspected, and a decision made about whether to repair or replace it. If the valve is to be replaced it is excised; the posterior leaflet is often left in place as there is considerable evidence that this improves left ventricular function. The valve is then sized and the appropriate replacement valve selected. The replacement is sewn into place, and a further 500 ml of cardioplegia is given as about 30 minutes will have elapsed. If the mitral valve has been repaired and tested, at least a further 500 ml bolus of cardioplegia is given. A patient with mitral stenosis would have a valvotomy where a patient with combined stenosis and regurgitation or regurgitation alone would have a more complex procedure. Finally the left atrium is closed and the patient rewarmed. After the left atrium has been closed the air is removed from the heart and the aortic cross–clamp is released, allowing the heart to reperfuse. If sinus rhythm does not return spontaneously then defibrillation, or pacing, or both, are undertaken until a satisfactory cardiac action is achieved. The patient is weaned from bypass, the atrial cannulas removed, and the heparin reversed with protamine. The aortic cannula is removed and after haemostasis has been secured, the chest is closed.

The operative mortality in the United Kingdom for isolated first time mitral valve replacement in 1990 was 5.2% for mechanical prostheses, 7.3% for xenograft replacement, and 0.9% for mitral valve repair. These figures do not differentiate between operations for mitral stenosis and mitral regurgitation.

Tricuspid stenosis

Tricuspid stenosis, like mitral stenosis, is almost always caused by rheumatic fever, and rarely occurs without rheumatic changes to the mitral valve. It can occur as a result of rheumatic disease of the aortic valve without involvement of the mitral valve, but this is rare. The pathological processes are similar to those that occur in the mitral valve. Tricuspid stenosis may also be associated with carcinoid disease, in which case there is a cicatricial deformity with commissural fusion and thickening and fusion of the chordae tendineae with thickening and shortening of the leaflets. Tricuspid regurgitation often coexists with tricuspid stenosis. Operation is rarely indicated for pure tricuspid stenosis unless the right atrial pressures are considerably raised and the patient has hepatic congestion, pleural effusions, ascites, and peripheral oedema.

Tricuspid regurgitation

The aetiology of tricuspid regurgitation is similar to that of mitral regurgitation, and it can occur as a result of disease of the annulus, of the leaflet tissue, or of the tensioning apparatus. Annular dilatation can occur in an anatomically normal valve as a consequence of right ventricular dilatation. In patients with rheumatic mitral valve disease it is not uncommon for the tricuspid regurgitation to result from secondary pulmonary hypertension and right ventricular dilatation rather than a rheumatic process itself. Rheumatic tricuspid valve disease is similar to rheumatic mitral valve disease, with commissural fusion, leaflet fibrosis and thickening, and chordal shortening and fusion.

Operation is rarely indicated for solitary tricuspid regurgitation, though repair or replacement of the valve may be indicated in conjunction with mitral valve surgery.

Surgery of the tricuspid valve

The chest is opened through a standard median sternotomy and the heart exposed. Heparin is given and the heart cannulated for cardiopulmonary bypass. The ascending aorta is cannulated to allow space to place an aortic cross–clamp and if necessary a cardioplegia cannula. The right atrium is cannulated with two venous cannulas, one placed through the atrial appendage and into the superior vena cava, the other through a separate atrial purse string and into the inferior vena cava, after which bypass is begun. The superior vena cava and inferior vena cava are then enclosed within tapes and snuggers which are tightened to exclude the heart completely from the venous system. Assuming that there is not a patent foramen ovale or any other intracardiac right to left connections it is now possible to open the right atrium without the aorta being cross–clamped and with the body temperature being maintained near normal. More usually the heart is fibrillated electrically before the atrium is opened so that the atrial septum can be inspected to exclude an intracardiac shunt. Alternatively the aorta can be cross–clamped, the patient cooled, and cardioplegia given in the standard fashion.

The right atrium is opened with a vertical incision and the tricuspid valve is exposed and inspected; one then decides whether to repair or replace it. If the valve is to be replaced then it is excised. The replacement valve is then sized and the appropriate one selected. Alternatively the tricuspid valve is repaired and tested. Finally the right atrium is closed, the patient is rewarmed, and air is removed from the heart. The caval snuggers are released and the patient is weaned from bypass. The atrial cannulas are removed and the heparin reversed with protamine. The aortic cannula is removed and after haemostasis has been fully secured, the chest is closed.

The operative mortality in the United Kingdom for isolated first time tricuspid valve replacement or repair in 1990 was 17.4%, although this was based on only 23 cases. The mortality for patients having first time multiple valve replacements that included a tricuspid valve procedure was about 15%, based on only 121 patients. These figures do not differentiate between operations for tricuspid stenosis and tricuspid regurgitation.

Pulmonary valve disease

Adult presentation of congenital pulmonary stenosis is rare, and treatment is usually by percutaneous balloon dilatation. Pulmonary regurgitation is well tolerated by the right ventricle and replacement of the pulmonary valve is rare.

Endocarditis

Native valve endocarditis

Indications for surgery

Patients with native valve endocarditis will be managed medically, with intravenous antibiotics and treatment for heart failure. If the medical treatment is successful they will subsequently have their valvar damage assessed at the appropriate time. The indications for early operation include evidence of uncontrolled infection while on appropriate antibiotics, worsening heart failure, or uncontrollable heart failure at presentation.

Only a few of the 6000 patients a year who have heart valves replaced, including repeat operations with or without associated coronary artery surgery, are operated on for acute native valve endocarditis. The overall caseload is probably less than 200 patients/year.

The patients referred for urgent operations are failing to respond to medical treatment, and are therefore expected to die without operation.

Patients operated on with active native valve endocarditis are at a higher risk than if their valve has been sterilised by antibiotic treatment. Under these circumstances valve replacement, or repair, is then being undertaken electively for the complications of endocarditis such as valvar regurgitation and heart failure. There is a considerably increased risk of prosthetic valve endocarditis developing in patients who are operated on for native valve endocarditis compared with non-infective valve disease. It is partly for this reason, and partly because these patients have infective lesions at the time of operation as well as an increased incidence of renal failure, that their operative risk is increased. As their chances of surviving without operation are small, however, they still gain considerable benefit from operation. The most important thing is to predict early that medical treatment is failing, and then to operate before their condition deteriorates further.

Operation of valve replacement for endocarditis

Under cardiopulmonary bypass and with the heart arrested, the heart is opened, the native valve is removed, and the annulus debrided. Extensive efforts are made to remove any infected material, and abscess cavities are obliterated. The choice of valve depends on the operating surgeon's preference, and a Starr-Edwards valve may be chosen because its sewing ring conforms easily to the annulus, particularly if the annulus is distorted by infection. Many surgeons will implant their favoured valve without further discussion, while others believe that the superior resistance to endocarditis of a homograft valve makes this the valve of choice in spite of the increased technical difficulty of implantation. The question of the possible increased resistance to endocarditis of xenografts compared with mechanical valves, balanced by the increased durability of mechanical valves, remains unresolved.

After operation all these patients will require prolonged courses of intravenous antibiotics, together with careful follow up. The development of signs of prosthetic valve endocarditis or heart failure whilst receiving appropriate intravenous antibiotics is particularly worrying, and inevitably leads to further operation with the same or a higher risk.

Prosthetic valve endocarditis

Prosthetic valve endocarditis is a dreaded complication of replacement valve surgery as only about half the patients survive in the long term. It is difficult to give an estimate of the risk as most published series are small, but an estimate of 1–2% is probably justified. Not surprisingly, the risk is increased by a factor of five if the operation is for native valve endocarditis. Lesser risk factors include prolonged duration of the original operation. This presumably reflects the increased duration of exposure of the valve to potential surface contamination during implantation. There is probably a slightly increased risk during the early period with mechanical valves and a lower risk with homografts, with xenografts between the two; but the published data are weak.

The aetiology of prosthetic valve endocarditis is different depending on the length of time that has elapsed between the initial operation and the onset of the endocarditis. Prosthetic valve endocarditis that develops within three to six months of the initial operation is caused by contamination at the initial operation, or from bacteraemia resulting from careless handling of intravenous cannulas during the early postoperative period. Endocarditis that develops after this period is generally a new event and caused by bacteraemia associated with dental, urological, or other instrumentation. This is supported by the findings that prosthetic valve endocarditis in the early phase is usually caused by staphylococci, Gram negative cocci or mixed organisms, whereas the organisms involved in late prosthetic valve endocarditis tend to be streptococci. Fungal infections are particularly devastating, and most patients who develop them will die.

In the United Kingdom, about 4200 first time valve replacement operations a year are done at present, implanting a total of about 4900 valves. If there was a 1.5% risk/operation of early prosthetic valve endocarditis this would produce about 65 cases/year. Patients present with general malaise, low grade fevers of unknown origin, symptoms of heart failure, signs of severe sepsis, or any combination of these. They will usually, but not necessarily have combinations of splinter haemorrhages, conjunctival or palatal petechiae, Roth's spots in the retina, and microscopic haematuria. Splenic infarcts, with pain and enlargement may occur, and with severe prosthetic valve endocarditis septic emboli and infarction can be widespread. Anaemia is common. Finding a paraprosthetic leak will confirm the diagnosis. An occasional patient will be lucky enough to have early bacteriological cure by antibiotics before a paraprosthetic leak develops, but these are in a minority, and most patients will require reoperation. The usual strategy is to treat the patients with a prolonged course of the appropriate antibiotic before reoperating. Unfortunately reoperation is often precipitated earlier than either the surgeon or cardiologist would wish by uncontrolled infection or worsening heart failure.

Untreated, the disease generally progresses to heart failure, resulting from

---

Signs of early prosthetic valve endocarditis

- Malaise
- Severe infection
- Anaemia
- Petechiae, microscopic haematuria
- Low grade fever
- Heart failure
- Splinter haemorrhages

dehiscence of the valve from the annulus, overwhelming sepsis, and death. If one is forced into operating by the deteriorating clinical course, the risk of the operation is increased but the alternative is certain death. For this group of patients risks have to be estimated individually. The operation is often a salvage procedure, and so the risks are generally irrelevant, but more important is the understanding that the risks rise sharply the longer the patient fails to respond to medical treatment. It is imperative that the patient's case is discussed with the appropriate surgical team so that the operation can be done at the optimal time. A moribund patient referred from a peripheral hospital after a prolonged and failing course of antibiotic treatment for prosthetic valve (or even native valve) endocarditis is worryingly common.

The operative risk for repeat valve surgery is about twice that of the initial operation. The overall risk for all first time single valve surgery in the United Kingdom is about 4.6%, and for all repeat single valve surgery about 8.6%. Operating in the presence of infection increases the risks, and probably many that die after single valve surgery are doing so after surgery for native valve endocarditis. Because only a proportion of those having repeat valve surgery are having it for endocarditis, we can speculate that the operative risk alone for prosthetic valve endocarditis is probably about 20%, and this is in line with the evidence that only about half the patients with prosthetic valve endocarditis will survive in the long term.

Valve replacement for prosthetic valve endocarditis

The technique of valve replacement for prosthetic valve endocarditis is essentially the same as for prosthetic valve failure. Under cardiopulmonary bypass and with the heart arrested, the heart is opened, the old valve is removed, and the annulus debrided. Extensive efforts are made to remove any infected material, and abscess cavities are obliterated. The choice of valve depends on the operating surgeon's preference. As for native valve endocarditis, a Starr-Edwards valve may be chosen because of the ease with which its sewing ring conforms to the annulus. Many surgeons will simply reimplant their favoured valve, and others believe that the superior resistance of a homograft valve to endocarditis makes it the valve of choice despite the difficulty of implanting it.

Prosthetic valve dysfunction and failure

About 15% of all valve operations done in the United Kingdom are repeat operations. The overall number of repeat operations is likely (certainly in the short to medium term), to climb, but the proportion of repeat operations to initial operations will fall. This is explained by the increasing trend to implant mechanical valves as opposed to tissue valves (xenograft or biological) at the first operation, and the time before tissue valves fail.

Most reoperations for failure of tissue valves are for gradual degeneration;

stenosis and incompetence develop as the valves calcify, or tear, or both. Tissue valve failure is usually a gradual process, allowing the patients to undergo reassessment and reoperation. This group of patients are not emergencies, but it is clear that a small number do present acutely with symptoms of sudden failure of the tissue valve. This generally results from sudden tearing of one of the cusps of a tissue valve, which leaves the valve acutely and severely incompetent. Our experience is that sudden failure is an under appreciated mode of failure of tissue valves, and is often diagnosed late. Sudden failure of mechanical valves, such as leaflet escape or strut fracture, is well recognised but unusual.

Patients with catastrophic prosthetic valve failure are often in cardiogenic shock at presentation or develop it rapidly. Without operation they are likely to die, so operation is indicated despite the increased risks. The overall risks of reoperation for valve replacement are about twice those of the initial operation, but the results are based on the data for all operations done. For the subgroup of patients with catastrophic prosthetic valve failure the risks are probably 25–40%, though there are few data.

Prosthetic valve replacement

Many of these patients will be intubated and ventilated before their transfer to theatre. For prosthetic mitral valve failure an intra–aortic balloon pump can be helpful, it is absolutely contraindicated in aortic regurgitation. Bypass will often be instituted through femoral artery and vein cannulation, which allows re-entry through the sternum and dissection of the heart from the adhesions to be done more safely. With the heart arrested, it is opened, the old valve is removed, the annulus debrided, and the new valve inserted.

Most surgeons would insert a mechanical valve under these circumstances, but some argue that a tissue valve should be inserted if that type would usually be appropriate for the age and requirements of the particular patient.

Postoperative management of valvar heart disease

Antibiotic prophylaxis

Any patient who has an abnormal valve or has had a valve replacement must be warned of the risks of endocarditis and should have antibiotic prophylaxis before dental treatment, or any other procedure that has potential to cause bacteraemia. The current recommendations for adults are given in the boxes.

Warfarin

All patients with mechanical prostheses must be treated with warfarin for life. Patients with homograft or xenograft aortic valves do not require

Dental procedures under local or no anaesthesia

- Including those with a prosthetic valve (but not endocarditis) who have *not* had any penicillin during the previous month:
  Amoxycillin 3 g orally one hour before
- Including those with a prosthetic valve (but not endocarditis) who *have* had penicillin during the previous month *or* who are allergic to penicillin:
  Clindamycin 600 mg orally one hour before
- Those who have had endocarditis:
  Amoxycillin 1 g (intramuscularly or intravenously) *plus* gentamicin 120 mg intravenously at induction *plus* amoxycillin 500 mg orally six hours later

warfarin, although some units give it for the first six to twelve weeks. Patients with xenograft mitral valves in sinus rhythm, with no evidence of thrombo-embolic disease, and in whom the left atrial appendage has been obliterated do not require long term warfarin, although again some units give it for the first six to twelve weeks. Most patients who have mitral valve replacement will be in atrial fibrillation, however, and for this reason alone should be anticoagulated, so it is sensible to implant mechanical valves into this group.

Dental procedures under general anaesthesia

- Those at no special risk (including those who have not had any penicillin during the previous month):
  Either amoxycillin 1 g (intravenously or intramuscularly) at induction, then amoxycillin 500 mg orally six hours later
  Or amoxycillin 3 g orally plus probenecid 1 g four hours before
- Those with a prosthetic valve or who have had endocarditis:
  Amoxycillin 1 g (intramuscularly or intravenously) *plus* gentamicin 120 mg intravenously at induction *plus* amoxycillin 500 mg orally six hours later
- Those who have had penicillin during the previous month *plus* who are allergic to penicillin:
  Either vancomycin 1 g infused over at least 100 minutes plus gentamicin 120 mg at induction
  Or teicoplanin 400 mg *plus* gentamicin 120 mg intravenously at induction
  Or clindamycin 300 mg given over at least 10 minutes at induction *plus* clindamycin 150 mg orally or intramuscularly six hours later

Other procedures

- Upper respiratory tract:
  As for dental procedures
- Genitourinary:
  As for those with prosthetic valves or who have had endocarditis, dental procedures. Clindamycin should not be given. If urine is infected, the organism should be treated
- Obstetric, gynaecological, and gastrointestinal:
  Prophylaxis is required only for patients with prosthetic valves or who have had endocarditis. Clindamycin should not be given, but any infecting organism should be treated

The recommended international normalised ratio (INR) seems to vary, but patients with higher INRs have a lower incidence of thromboembolic complications but a higher incidence of bleeding complications. The target INR varies with the type of prosthetic valve inserted; an INR of 2.5–3.0 for aortic prostheses and 3.0–3.5 for mitral prostheses is not uncommon. It has been suggested that the addition of an antiplatelet agent such as aspirin may permit a lower INR.

Appendix: Anatomy of the cardiac valves

The interior of the left ventricle contains a number of structures, including the orifices of its two valves. The left atrioventricular or mitral orifice which is oval lies below and slightly to the left of the aortic orifice, which is circular.

The mitral valve has two leaflets, anterior and posterior. The anterior or septal leaflet is the larger, and is roughly triangular with its base inserting over about a third of the mitral annulus. The smaller posterior leaflet inserts over about two thirds of the annulus and its free edge is usually described as scalloped, whereas the anterior leaflet has a smooth free edge. The anterior cusp is 15–18 mm long, and the posterior 10–12 mm, so when the valve is closed there is a large area of coaptation of the leaflets. The leaflets are supported by chordae tendineae, cordis, which are fibrous bands that pass to the two large papillary muscles of the left ventricle, the anterolateral and the posteromedial papillary muscles. Each leaflet receives chordae tendineae from both papillary muscles, most inserting on the free leaflet edge. Three orders of chordae have been defined; the first order inserts on the free edge of the leaflet, and the second order some millimetres back from the free edge. The third order applies only to the posterior leaflet where some chordae attach to the base of the leaflet.

The aortic valve is usually tricuspid, made up of a fibrous skeleton, shaped like a crown. This skeleton is continuous with the anterior leaflet of the mitral valve and the membranous septum. Suspended from the skeleton are the three fibrous cusps, commonly called the left, right, and non-coronary cusps because of their relation to the orifices of the coronary arteries. At the midpoint of the free edge of each cusp is a fibrous nodule, the nodules of Arantius, and on either side of each nodule is a thin crescent shaped portion of the cusp, the lunula. The lunula together with the nodules of Arantius form the area of coaptation of the valve during its closure.

There are two valves associated with the right ventricle, the inlet atrioventricular (or tricuspid) valve, and the outlet pulmonary valve. The tricuspid valve, as its name suggests, has three leaflets, the anterior, posterior, and septal. The septal leaflet is related to the interventricular septum, and the anterior leaflet runs between the septum and the infundibulum. The pulmonary valve has three cusps, two sited anteriorly, one to the right and one to the left, and the third is situated posteriorly.

8 Surgical options in the management of heart and lung failure

- Acute heart failure
- Chronic heart failure
    Cardiac transplantation
    Cardiomyoplasty
- Acute pulmonary and cardiopulmonary failure
- Chronic cardiopulmonary and pulmonary failure
    Cardiopulmonary transplantation
    Pulmonary transplantation
- Postoperative management of patients with transplants
    Immunosuppression

Introduction

There are a number of surgical options in the management of heart and lung failure, and these can be divided into acute and chronic.

Surgical management of acute heart failure depends mostly on the intra–aortic balloon pump, though experience is increasing in the use of various blood pumps to support the circulation until the patient recovers or a donor organ becomes available. In certain cases the native heart can be replaced with a totally implanted artificial heart as a temporary measure before transplantation.

At present the only effective treatment for chronic failure of these organs is

---

Decision making in cardiac and pulmonary failure

- Heart failure, lung failure, or both?
- Acute or chronic?
- Recoverable or irreversible?
    If recoverable, suitable for support to recovery?
    If irreversible, suitable for transplantation?
- Most appropriate technique?

---

orthotopic allograft transplantation — that is, transplantation of a donor organ of the same species into the same site after excision of the native organ. Totally implanted artificial hearts have, so far, been unsuccessful as long term implants in chronic heart failure, though work is continuing. There is considerable interest and progress being made in the use of paracorporeal blood pumps to support the heart in chronic heart failure, and these may turn out to be more effective in the long term than a totally implanted artificial heart. Xenotransplantation has been attempted a few times, but so far without success. Cardiomyoplasty, a new technique which uses the patient's own muscle to support the heart, is controversial. At present there is little progress in methods of chronic lung support other than transtracheal oxygen supply devices.

Acute heart failure

Intra-aortic balloon pump

The intra-aortic balloon pump was first developed in the 1960s to provide mechanical support to a failing heart. In addition to its mechanical action, and possibly more importantly, it improves coronary blood flow in diastole.

Indications

Intra-aortic balloon pumping may be used either as support while the patient waits for an operation, or as part of the treatment of postoperative cardiogenic shock. Patients for whom it is suitable preoperatively have either a mechanical lesion that is amenable to operation, including severe unstable angina, mitral regurgitation after infarction, and ventricular septal rupture after infarction (otherwise known as "postinfarction ventricular septal defect"). These patients will have had Swan-Ganz catheters inserted and be receiving inotropic support, and despite this still have cardiogenic shock.

Balloon pumping for postoperative cardiogenic shock is usually started in the operating theatre when there is difficulty in weaning patients from cardiopulmonary bypass. These patients will also be given inotropic support,

---

Cardiogenic shock

- Low cardiac index (cardiac output/body surface area) with adequate filling pressures
- For example: index < 2 l/m^2
  plus central venous pressure > 15 mmHg
  plus left atrial pressure > 20 mmHg

---

and will usually have had Swan-Ganz catheters already in place because they are the patients in the higher risk groups. If not, they can be managed, at least during the early period, by direct measurement of left atrial and pulmonary artery pressures with pressure measuring catheters placed directly while the chest is open.

Mechanism of action

The intra-aortic balloon pump used in adults is a 34 ml or 40 ml balloon (depending on patient size) filled with helium that is positioned in the descending thoracic aorta just distal to the left subclavian artery. It is connected by a long polyethylene cannula through a femoral artery to a bedside console. The console pumps the helium in and out of the balloon according to the program chosen. The volume to which the balloon is inflated (up to a maximum of 40 ml), the delay between the R-wave and balloon inflation, and the duration of balloon inflation can all be varied. The frequency with which cardiac cycles are supported (from every cycle to only 1 in 10), can also be varied. The balloon is usually set to fill to 40 ml; the start of filling coincides with closure of the aortic valve in diastole and the pump is actively emptied in presystole. The effect is to transfer energy into the blood stream during diastole, forcing a wave of pressure in a retrograde direction and increasing coronary perfusion during diastole, while the active emptying in presystole (late diastole) allows the heart to eject into a reduced aortic pressure (fig 8.1). This reduces the afterload, and allows the heart to consume less energy to eject the same volume of blood.

Insertion

The intra-aortic balloon pump can be inserted in several ways, but the simplest is by the Seldinger technique. A needle is inserted into the femoral artery, and a guide wire placed through the needle before the needle is withdrawn. Either a dilator and then an introducer sheath can be inserted over the guide wire or, with newer models, the balloon pump itself can be introduced directly over the guide wire without an introducer sheath. The alternative approach is to expose the common femoral artery through a cut down, and to insert the balloon pump either directly through a small stab

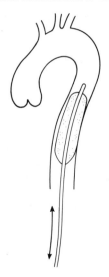

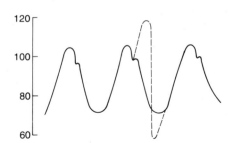

Figure 8.1 The technique of insertion of the intra-aortic balloon. The balloon is shown inflated in the descending aorta. The pressure trace shows augmentation in diastole together with the reduction in pressure in late diastole (the pre-systolic dip).

incision in the artery, or by the Seldinger technique under direct vision. Either local or general anaesthesia can be used.

On the rare occasions where neither of these techniques is appropriate and the chest is open, the balloon pump can be inserted directly through the ascending aorta and passed down the aorta rather than up it.

Removal

The pump is usually removed by the route through which it is inserted. A percutaneous pump is removed and pressure is placed over the entry site (into the artery, rather than over the exit site from the skin which may be some centimetres away), and a pump which was inserted through a cut down may be removed through a further cut down. In some units an elective femoral embolectomy is done at the time that the pump is removed, and so the pump will always be removed through a cut down.

Ventricular assist devices

A few patients have such poor cardiac function that even multiple inotropes, phosphodiesterase inhibitors, and vasodilators, together with the balloon pump will not keep them alive. Increasingly consideration is given to the use of mechanical devices to support their circulation, either as support until cardiac function recovers or as a temporary measure while waiting for transplantation. Most assist devices consist of sacks containing blood in which a rigid chamber is separated into two parts by a flexible membrane. On one side of the membrane the unidirectional flow of blood is maintained through inlet and outlet valves similar to the normal ventricle, and on the other side of the membrane is a system that displaces the membrane, and pumps blood through the chamber. This effect can be achieved either by pumping compressed air in and out or by using an electrically driven mechanical device to push against the membrane. The main complications of these devices include bleeding, renal failure, stroke, and mediastinitis.

Indications

The two ventricles should be considered as separate functional entities, even though right ventricular dysfunction may be secondary to left ventricular failure. Either ventricle may need independent assistance or both ventricles may require support simultaneously. Left ventricular assistance is considered when the patient is being treated with inotropic infusions and an intra-aortic balloon pump and the left atrial pressure is still above 25 mmHg, the systolic blood pressure less than 90 mmHg, and the cardiac index less than 1.6 l/min/m^2. Right ventricular assistance is considered when the right atrial pressure is above 25 mmHg and the left atrial pressure is low, with a cardiac index less than 1.6 l/min/m^2.

Insertion and removal

Ventricular assist devices are inserted at sternotomy, and often require cardiopulmonary bypass support because the heart has to be manipulated for cannulation. The exact technique of cannulation depends on the device used, but usually right ventricular support consists of right atrial drainage and pulmonary artery return, and left ventricular support consists of either left atrial or left ventricular drainage and ascending aortic return. After weaning from ventricular assist, removal procedure is the reverse of the insertion procedure.

Other systems

Patients can be supported for a short time with a normal bypass circuit, though it is not safe to do this for more than about 12 hours. The performance of the circuit can be improved by avoiding the use of an oxygenator whenever possible, and by using constrained vortex pumps rather than roller pumps. A new system is the "haemopump", in which an Archimedes screw arrangement is used, with a catheter passing from the left ventricle to the descending aorta. Within the catheter is a small impeller, which is rotated at high speed (30 000 rpm) by a cable driven from an external console. This drives blood from the left ventricle into the aorta. The role of this system is yet to be established, and for the moment it remains an investigational device.

Chronic heart failure

Underlying diseases

There are a number of conditions that have a common end point in heart failure, either acute or chronic. Acute heart failure can be precipitated by myocardial infarction, viral illnesses, and by drugs. Chronic heart failure usually results from ischaemic heart disease, but can also develop after a viral infection. In many younger patients heart failure is labelled "cardiomyopathy", because no precipitating cause can be identified.

Natural history of congestive heart failure

Data on the annual incidence of congestive heart failure is based on long term prospective studies of large populations, and the Framingham study of 5209 subjects followed up for more than 30 years showed initial evidence of cardiac failure developing in 461 men and women. The average annual incidence increased from 3/1000 at the ages of 35–64 years to 10/1000 at the ages of 65–94 years.

Data from the same study showed that, assuming that there was not a correctable mechanical problem, overt heart failure is lethal. Within two years of its diagnosis, 37% of men and 38% of women had died, and during six years of follow up the mortality was 82% for men and 67% for women. Review of data from the National Center for Health Statistics in the United States suggests that in 1983, 33 227 deaths were ascribed to congestive heart failure. Congestive heart failure was given as a secondary cause of death on a further 160 000 death certificates.

The most recent figures for England and Wales suggest that about 200 000 people die each year in the United Kingdom for whom "heart disease" is given as the cause of death. These are extremely crude figures, and it is difficult to clarify the underlying conditions, but many of them will have died in left ventricular failure caused by ischaemic heart disease. Compared with the figures from the United States, it would be predicted that the annual death rate in the United Kingdom from congestive heart failure would be 10 000–12 000 a year.

In a study undertaken before angiotensin converting enzyme inhibitors were used, reported survival rates were 66% at 12 months, 41% at 24 months, and 24% at 36 months. The authors pointed out that cardiac index, stroke volume, and stroke work were all significantly lower in those who died. Some of the best recent data comes from the consensus study, in which treatment with an angiotensin converting enzyme inhibitor was compared with a placebo added to the conventional treatment that the patients were already receiving. Though there was a reduction in crude mortality of 40% at six months in the treated group compared with the placebo, the overall mortality was 44% in the placebo group and 26% in the treated group at six months. This benefit reflects the reduction in mortality from congestive heart failure, there being no reduction in the mortality from sudden death.

When symptoms, and in particular measures of exercise tolerance, start to worsen in an otherwise stable patient, that is the time to intervene. There is evidence, however, that patients with severely depressed ejection fraction ($<20\%$), or stroke volume (<40 ml), or both; severe dysrhythmia (resuscitated ventricular fibrillation or sustained ventricular tachycardia); and a pronounced rise in the plasma noradrenaline concentration (>800 pg/ml), are at particular and imminent risk of death. This is confirmed by studies that identified pulmonary artery wedge capillary pressure at rest and peak exercise stroke work index as independent predictors of mortality.

Cardiac transplantation

The first documented successful attempts at experimental cardiac transplantation were by Carrel and Guthrie in 1905, who transplanted hearts into heterotopic positions in dogs. During the early 1940s Demikhov in the USSR did an extensive series of experimental cardiac transplantation procedures in dogs but only relatively recently has his work become known. It was not until the advent of cardiopulmonary bypass techniques, however, that serious progress could be made.

The first successful experimental orthotopic transplants in dogs were reported by Lower and Shumway in 1960, and the first cardiac transplant into a human was done in 1964 when Hardy used a baboon heart in a desperate attempt to save a patient in cardiogenic shock. This attempt was unsuccessful as the graft failed within an hour of implantation from hyperacute rejection.

This attempt, although not widely publicised, was the first of a small number of xenotransplants, the use of which declined as allotransplantation

111

increased. It has been reported that other groups used porcine hearts to try to save patients who could not be weaned from cardiopulmonary bypass at the end of operations, but these attempts also failed. Recently with the increasing incidence of mismatch between donors and recipients there has been an increase in experimental activity, but for the moment the prospects of successful clinical xenotransplantation are still some way off.

While Shumway at Stanford and Kantrowitz in New York continued their experimental work in allotransplantation, Barnard in Cape Town did the first successful cardiac transplant in a human, late in 1967. This generated an enormous amount of publicity, and was followed by an explosion of interest in cardiac transplantation, a large number of transplant operations, and an almost equally large number of medium to long term failures.

This almost complete lack of success, mainly the result of the difficulties of balancing effective control of rejection against excessive immunosuppression and overwhelming infection, quickly led to an almost universal abandonment of cardiac transplantation. The major exception was at Stanford where Shumway continued an experimental and clinical programme at a steady pace. His continuing success meant that clinical cardiac transplantation gradually became accepted again during the late 1970s and early 1980s, and the number of procedures increased in the mid 1980s, particularly as the use of cyclosporin A became widespread. Cardiac transplantation has now increased to such a point that the main limiting factor is the mismatch between the relatively few donor organs and the number of suitable recipients.

Indications for cardiac transplantation

At present only around 350 hearts are available each year in the United Kingdom and the gap between demand for transplantation and the supply of organs is likely to increase. The mismatch is worse in the United States where in 1988 it was estimated that there were about 14 000 potential candidates for transplantation, and about 1000 donor organs available. With evidence that older patients do well after transplantation and the increasing pressure from an ageing society to treat older patients in general, the mismatch between the number of available organs and potential donors is likely to increase still further. Efforts to increase the preservation time continue with a view to widening the catchment area for donors around any one centre, but it is inevitable that the increasing use of donor organs in areas that have not previously had transplant units but have supplied organs, negates the benefits of the increased preservation time.

In theory any patient with heart failure and without other organ disease, evidence of malignancy, or overwhelming sepsis is a candidate for cardiac transplantation. In real terms though there is an age range, and though the bottom end of the age range is down to well under 1 year of age in the United Kingdom, the upper age limit is currently about 60 years of age. There is

---

Intra–aortic balloon pump

Indications

- Low cardiac output after cardiac surgery
- Preoperatively
  Acute ventricular septal rupture
  Acute mitral regurgitation after infarction
  Awaiting cardiac transplantation

Contraindications

- Aortic regurgitation
- Severe peripheral vascular disease

---

some variation between different units, but it is unusual for a patient more than 60 years old to receive a transplant. Unfortunately because of the system by which organs are offered for transplantation it is not possible to prioritise among patients nationally but only within any one unit.

There are contraindications to transplantation, some of which are absolute and others which are relative, and these are shown in the boxes. If for example, the renal or hepatic impairment was acute or clearly secondary to cardiac failure and one expected that it would be reversed by improving the cardiac output, then it would be less of a contraindication to transplantation. Occasionally heart transplantation has been combined with renal transplantation, but this is unusual.

Risks and benefits of the operation

For those patients who are lucky enough to receive a transplant, there is, even in the most experienced centres, at best a five year survival of about 80%. In 1989, the most recent period for which worldwide figures are available, operative mortality was 10% in orthotopic heart transplantation, with a current one year survival of 81% for adults and an actuarial five year

---

Absolute contraindications to transplantation

- Cancer within five years
- Other end-stage organ failure
- Overwhelming sepsis
- AIDS
- Tuberculosis
- Aspergillosis
- Dementia

Relative contraindications to transplantation

- Hepatitis B or C infection
- Moderate renal or hepatic impairment
- Evidence of non-compliance with treatment
- Psychosocial instability

survival of 72%. These figures are worse for children, with a five year actuarial survival of 62%. The primary difference between children and adults is the higher operative mortality in the youngest recipients, but even in adults most of the deaths within the first year occur during the first two weeks. Reasons include multiple organ failure, acute graft dysfunction, early rejection, overwhelming infection, and major bleeding. As for any other type of cardiac surgery, cerebral damage and acute renal failure may also contribute to early postoperative death.

The risk benefit analysis must balance risks of morbidity and mortality against the potential improvements in symptoms and prognosis. The risk of dying from congestive heart failure reaches about 75% at 36 months for a patient receiving medical treatment. Confirmation that this estimate is reasonable comes from other data that suggest that between 25% and 30% of patients accepted on to a waiting list for transplantation will die before a suitable donor becomes available.

Data about survival after transplantation indicate that a patient for whom a suitable donor organ is found has a risk of about 25% of dying within three years of the operation. If we extend the analysis to five years, the risk of dying from congestive heart failure reaches about 95%, while the risk of dying after transplantation is relatively stable, having increased to only about 28%. If we take a 10 year view and allow a loss of 5% a year, then by 10 years after the operation we could expect that about half of those undergoing transplantation will still be alive, while all those with heart failure treated medically will have died. Obviously this analysis is somewhat premature, as the number of patients who have been operated on since 1980, and have had the chance to live for 10 years, is still low.

Examination of survival data gives an analysis of prognosis, but it bears no relation to the effect of the procedure on control of symptoms and a patient's ability to return to an acceptable lifestyle. This sort of information is a little harder to gather, but it is clear that many patients gain good control of their symptoms and are able to achieve lifestyles that are commensurate with those of their social peers. The chances of returning to work depend not only on a patient's occupation, but also on the length of the illness, and age. A younger patient who has had a short illness before transplantation has a better chance of returning to work than an older patient with chronic disease. There are, however, numerous examples of patients who have returned to highly active lifestyles after cardiac transplantation.

Clearly the more ill patients are before transplantation, the more potential benefit they have to gain. Against this is balanced a higher operative risk, with the potential loss of a donor heart. To decide whether an older but sicker patient with a high short term risk but higher medium term benefit should receive an organ rather than a younger, slightly fitter patient with a lower short term risk but not quite so pronounced medium term benefit can be difficult. With our increasing ability to maintain patients with severe heart failure on mechanical support devices the ethics of choice of recipient have the potential to become even more fraught.

The most important long term problem for patients who have received a heart transplant is the risk of accelerated graft atherosclerosis. The exact mechanism of this devastating complication is not clear, but the tubular narrowing of the coronary arteries of the donor ventricle produces silent myocardial ischaemia, with a gradual progression to worsening heart failure. Other long term complications include the development of renal failure from treatment with cyclosporin A, together with anaemia, hypertension, increased susceptibility to infection, and the development of lymphoproliferative disorders related to chronic immunosuppression.

Criteria of suitability of donors

The operation to implant the new heart is a small part of cardiac transplantation, and a number of events must happen before the operation can start. Once a potential donor has become available the suitability of the donor must be established. Brain stem death must have been established according to the widely recognised criteria. If the donor is male he should be under 50 years old, and a non-smoker. If the donor was a smoker then the upper age limit is lower (about 35 years of age) and for a female donor the age limit is usually about 10 years higher because of the lower incidence of coronary artery disease in women.

The cause of death must have been established, and there must be no evidence of infection, including hepatitis B and HIV, or of cancer, the exception to this being that confined to the brain. There should be no period of prolonged hypotension, no evidence of cardiac damage, and low doses of inotropes. It is important to realise that some of these contraindications are relative; an older donor with a potentially less suitable heart would be acceptable for an older recipient or a recipient who is unlikely to survive a wait for a better heart.

ABO compatibility and body size compatibility are then established, together with the appropriate operating theatre timings at the donor hospital. Where possible a recipient negative for cytomegalovirus should receive a heart from a donor who has not been exposed. A preliminary decision to proceed with donor harvest is then made and the appropriate harvesting

Criteria for donors

- Age: Male <50 years, female <60 years
- Non-smoker
- No previous history of cardiac disease or cancer
- Inotropic support less than 10 μg/kg/min of dopamine (or equivalent)
- ABO blood group compatible
- Similar exposure to cytomegalovirus as recipient
- Normal ECG (ST changes of sub-arachnoid haemorrhage may be acceptable)
- No prolonged hypotension or cardiac arrest
- No cardiac damage
- Central venous pressure <12 mmHg
- $PaO_2 > 100$ mmHg on FiO_2 of 0.4
- $PaCO_2 < 40$ mmHg at tidal volume of 15 ml/kg and ventilatory rate of 10–14/min

teams, implanting teams, theatre and anaesthetic personnel, and intensive care unit staff are alerted. If the potential recipient is not already in hospital, his or her whereabouts must be established and rapid transfer to the hospital organised. At the same time transport for the donor harvesting team to the donating hospital must be arranged, and the method of transfer will depend on the expected journey time.

On arrival at the donating hospital a further assessment of the donor's state is made before the heart is harvested. Assuming that it is satisfactory then the heart is removed in coordination with any groups harvesting other organs. Currently there is considerable interest in "optimising" the donor before removal of organs. This involves insertion of a pulmonary artery pressure catheter, with volume loading to wean the donor off inotropes such as adrenaline, or dobutamine. The idea is both to improve the quality of organs selected for donation, but also to try to resuscitate organs that at first sight do not look suitable for transplantation.

Harvesting the donor heart

A standard technique for donor harvesting is to divide the inferior vena cava at its passage through the diaphragm, to cross–clamp the aorta, and then give a cardioplegic solution into the aortic root. The left ventricle is then vented by dividing the right inferior pulmonary vein. After the cardioplegic solution has been given, the right superior pulmonary vein, both left pulmonary veins, and then the left and right pulmonary arteries are divided. The ascending aorta is then divided, and finally the superior vena cava, well clear of the right atrium and sinus node, after the central line has been removed.

The heart is then placed in a series of plastic bags, each filled with a litre of ice cold Hartmann's solution and placed into ice slush in an insulated box for transfer. Various cardioplegic solutions are used by different groups, but the ischaemic time should be kept under six hours, and preferably under four hours.

Removal of the diseased heart

The new heart is implanted on full cardiopulmonary bypass; the superior vena cava and inferior vena cava are cannulated separately, and the ascending aorta is cannulated. The cavas are occluded by snuggers, and the aorta cross–clamped.

The heart is excised with an incision that starts in the right atrial appendage, and passes down close to the atrioventricular groove to the origin of the coronary sinus. Incision in the coronary sinus allows the interatrial septum and free wall of the left atrium to be opened, and this incision is continued along the free wall of the left atrium in the left atrioventricular groove to the base of the left atrial appendage. Next the aorta and pulmonary artery are transected, and the incision along the atrial septum is completed. Finally the heart is excised by completing the division of the roof of the left atrium from the base of the left atrial appendage to the origin of the incision in the right atrial appendage.

Implanting the new heart

The donor heart is inspected for a patent foramen ovale, and if found this is oversewn. Incisions are made joining up the orifices of the pulmonary veins and excising the posterior wall of the left atrium. The right atrium is opened up with an incision running from the orifice of the inferior vena cava to the right atrial appendage.

The donor left atrial appendage is lined up to the site of the recipient left atrial appendage and a stitch is inserted superiorly for 2 or 3 cm. The other end of the stitch is run down towards the junction of the atrial septum, and the free walls of the left and right atria. Next the stitch is run along the left side of the recipient atrial septum, bringing it together with the left side of the donor atrial septum to join with the other end of the stitch, which now lies roughly below the pulmonary artery. The pulmonary arteries of recipient and donor are anastomosed, and then the aortas of recipient and donor are anastomosed. Implantation is completed with anastomosis of the two right atria, the stitch starting at the site of the donor right atrial appendage, after trimming of the recipient right atrial appendage. The stitch is run down the right side of the recipient atrial septum, bringing it together with the right side of the donor atrial septum. The free wall of the right atrium is then closed, and then the cut end of the donor superior vena cava is oversewn (see fig 8.2).

Air is removed and the aortic cross–clamp can be released and the heart

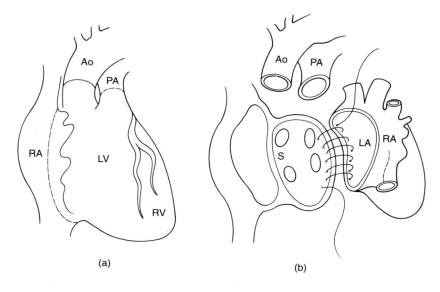

(a)

(b)

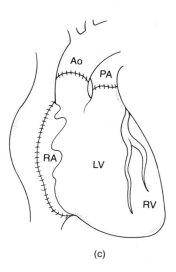

(c)

Figure 8.2 Cardiac transplantation. Both ventricles are excised leaving most of the atria behind. The left atrium (LA) of the donor heart, then the septum (S) and then the right atrium are sutured into position. The aorta (Ao) and the pulmonary artery (PA) are then sewn end to end.

reperfused. Extensive procedures to remove air are repeated and then the heart gradually weaned from bypass. A number of temporary pacing wires are left in, and the bypass cannulas are removed and the chest closed after haemostasis has been secured.

Cardiomyoplasty

Cardiomyoplasty is a new approach to the management of patients with chronic heart failure, and at present it is still experimental. We have included it here because it has the potential to be widely used in the treatment of heart failure in the medium to long term. The concept is that if skeletal muscle is subjected to repetitive electrical stimulation then a fast twitch, easily fatigued muscle can be converted to slow twitch, fatigue resistant muscle. This muscle can then be used to deliver chronic power.

Cardiomyoplasty requires the mobilisation of the latissimus dorsi muscle on its neurovascular pedicle, and it is applied to the heart as a method of mechanical support. In clinical practice it can be combined with other procedures, the most usual combination being with ventricular aneurysmectomy. It can, however, be done with valve replacement or repair, coronary artery bypass surgery, or (potentially) for the correction of congenital heart defects.

There has been extensive research into dynamic cardiomyoplasty but in contrast to cardiac transplantation, muscle powered counterpulsation devices, and skeletal muscle ventricles, dynamic cardiomyoplasty has come into clinical practice before some of the important experimental justification has been completed.

The early use of dynamic cardiomyoplasty in clinical practice reflects enthusiasm for the technique in certain centres, but its clinical assessment has been restricted by difficulties with logistics, cost, and consent and has mostly been confined to non-invasive methods. Evidence of success has been presented on clinical grounds and in the treatment of acute cardiac failure in animals, but only recently has evidence become available that it is effective in experimental chronic heart failure. There have also been reports of haemodynamic improvement in exercise tolerance in patients with moderately severe heart failure.

Indications for cardiomyoplasty

The conditions for which cardiomyoplasty will be considered are essentially the same as those for which orthotopic cardiac transplantation would be considered. The exception to this is Chagas' disease (South American trypanosomiasis) for which a number of cardiomyoplasties have been done in South America. There is a high risk of the disease developing in a donor heart, and so cardiomyoplasty without the immunosuppression of transplantation has potential advantages.

119

The patients for whom cardiomyoplasty is planned would have a similar life expectancy without operation as those awaiting transplantation.

Risks and benefits of the operation

Only a few patients have so far undergone cardiomyoplasty, but the initial data suggest in–hospital mortality of at least 10%, with an expected death rate amongst the survivors of about 5% a year. It must be emphasised that there have not yet been enough such operations done to construct actuarial survival curves.

This procedure is in the early phases of introduction into clinical practice at the time of writing, and it is too early to give accurate figures for its benefits. Currently about 50–100 patients a year undergo cardiomyoplasty and there are encouraging early clinical data that suggest that there are considerable benefits both in exercise tolerance and in survival. There are also experimental data that suggest that long term benefit is also to be expected.

The operation of cardiomyoplasty

Initially the patient is placed in a lateral position, with the left side up. A skin incision is made from the point of the scapula to the posterior superior iliac spine, and deepened down to the latissimus dorsi muscle. Skin flaps are reflected, both cranially and caudally, until the whole of the muscle has been released over its subcutaneous aspect. Next the anterior border and posterior borders are fully mobilised. The fibrous origin from the ribs is then divided and haemostasis on the chest wall and subcutaneous flaps secured. The mobilisation of the neurovascular pedicle is completed, and the tendon is divided close to the humerus.

The intercostal muscles over the second rib are divided and a 4 cm anterior arc of the second rib together with the periosteum is excised. The latissimus dorsi muscle is then passed into the chest through this space. Pacing leads are attached to the muscle and also passed into the chest. The chest wound is then closed, the patient placed supine, and a median sternotomy is made. The muscle is retrieved from the chest and passed around the heart, usually from posterior to anterior as a clockwise wrap when viewed from the apex of the heart. The muscle is secured in place by sutures to itself, in some places to the epicardium, and particularly to the pericardium. After insertion of the cardiomyostimulator the chest is closed. After a two week period to allow the muscle's blood supply to recover from the trauma of handling, the muscle stimulation protocol is commenced, converting the muscle from its fast twitch type II fibres to slow twitch type I fibres. This gives mechanical assistance to the failing heart. The protocol in current use indicates that it takes 12 weeks before the muscle produces its maximum support and this remains one of the major limitations of the procedure. There is some evidence that the muscle conditioning protocol can be considerably amended to improve the rate and to reduce some of the loss of power that occurs during muscle transformation.

Operation for acute pulmonary and cardiopulmonary failure

At present there are only two options in the treatment of acute pulmonary failure; the first is the intravascular oxygenator (IVOX), and the second is extracorporeal membrane oxygenation with removal of carbon dioxide (ECMO/ECO$_2$R). The IVOX is a system of hollow fibres, arranged as a bundle, which is inserted through a femoral vein into the inferior vena cava and right atrium. The principle is that oxygen is sucked through the interior of the fibres, and as the oxygen diffuses out into the blood stream, carbon dioxide will diffuse into the fibres and be excreted. The preliminary evidence is that this does not provide enough gas exchange to be clinically useful. The principles behind ECMO and ECO$_2$R are to rest the lungs and allow healing. The available techniques range from full cardiopulmonary bypass circuits to systems whereby blood is withdrawn at comparatively low flow rates from one large vein, passed through a membrane oxygenator, and returned to the right atrium through another large vein. The idea is to remove carbon dioxide through the membrane oxygenator, and at the same time provide adequate arterial oxygen tensions by continuous insufflation of oxygen into the lungs at relatively low pressures and ventilatory rates. Neither of these systems are suitable for chronic pulmonary failure, but ECMO has proved useful in neonates, particularly those with respiratory distress.

Operations for chronic cardiopulmonary and pulmonary failure

Cardiopulmonary transplantation

Heart-lung transplantation developed from the need to treat patients who had either pulmonary hypertension secondary to primary cardiac disease, or primary lung conditions with or without secondary cardiac disease. The first heart and lung transplant was performed in 1968 by Cooley, Lillehei did a second in 1969, and Barnard a third in 1971. All these attempts failed, and there was then a lull until the 1980s when the procedure was reintroduced by Reitz. Part of the reason for the gap was that dogs were the favoured experimental model, and dogs have a powerful Hering-Breuer reflex, so cannot breathe with a denervated heart-lung block. This limitation was not overcome until primates were used for experimental procedures.

There has been an increasing tendency recently to use single or double lung transplantation rather than heart-lung transplantation in patients with

121

isolated pulmonary disease, and if this is not appropriate the recipient's own "normal" heart is used as a donor organ for another patient. This is known as a "domino procedure".

Indications

Conditions for which heart-lung transplantation is considered include, Eisenmenger's syndrome, congenital and acquired heart disease with pulmonary hypertension, cystic fibrosis, primary pulmonary hypertension, emphysema, and end-stage fibrotic lung disease. As part of the drive to increase the number of patients to benefit from each organ donation, there has been a trend during recent years to do more single lung transplants, and some patients who previously might have received heart-lung transplantation for end-stage lung disease are now receiving single lung transplants instead. This policy is under review as there is increasing evidence that patients with infective lung disease are not suitable for single lung transplantation, and those with primary pulmonary hypertension may also be unsuitable. Heart-lung transplantation is usually now considered only for patients with Eisenmenger's syndrome. If both lungs need transplantation then either double lung transplantation or bilateral single lung transplantation is used.

Currently about 30 heart-lung transplants are done each year in the United Kingdom, and about 200 a year throughout the world. These small numbers reflect not only the technical complexity of the operation and the generally poor supply of donor organs, but also the trend towards single and sequential single lung transplants where possible.

Patients selected for heart-lung transplantation should have diseases that are not amenable to lesser procedures, be under 50 years of age, and have no other organ disease, evidence of malignancy, or overwhelming infection. In particular they should be seronegative for hepatitis B and HIV and have no evidence of active tuberculosis or aspergillosis. They should require less than 10 mg a day of prednisolone. Occasionally heart-lung transplantation has been combined with hepatic transplantation (as in cystic fibrosis), or renal transplantation, but this is unusual.

It has been hard to assess accurately the natural history of patients awaiting heart-lung transplantation as the population is more heterogeneous than those awaiting heart transplantation alone, but recently predictive factors for patients with cystic fibrosis have been described. It is clear that acceptance on to a waiting list for heart-lung transplantation indicates a poor prognosis without operation. There are potentially far more patients suitable for and deserving of transplantation than there are available donors, and so by the time patients are accepted on to waiting lists they are already in a particularly high risk group. Many of those undergoing heart-lung transplantation are already in hospital awaiting operation, some are already being ventilated before operation, and only a few are admitted from home. Some patients with primary pulmonary hypertension are receiving long term treatment at home with prostacyclin intravenously to lower their pulmonary vascular resistance while awaiting transplantation.

Risks and benefits of the operation

The risk of heart-lung transplantation is considerably higher than for heart transplantation alone. Not only is the operative mortality higher, but there is also a higher death rate during the postoperative period. About 70% of patients will be alive at one year, but by five years only about 40% will still be alive. Much of the early mortality is caused by the high incidence of excessive bleeding in the immediate postoperative period (particularly in those patients with scarring from previous thoracic surgery) and its associated complications. The late fall in survival is caused by the development of obliterative bronchiolitis in the transplanted lungs; sometimes this can be arrested by increasing the doses of antirejection drugs, but it is usually fatal without retransplantation.

It is clear that patients who survive a heart-lung transplant have good symptomatic control, but this will deteriorate if obliterative bronchiolitis develops. Though only 40% are alive at five years, without transplantation few would be expected to survive that long. As new antirejection drugs are developed, the proportion of the transplanted group alive at five years will increase, and this will eventually be reflected in the long term survival figures as well.

The operation of heart-lung transplantation

As for orthotopic heart transplantation, there is a considerable amount of planning that must go into setting up each heart-lung transplant operation, and the same type of assessments must be made. Ideally every donor should be considered initially as a heart-lung donor and if the lungs are not suitable as a heart donor alone. The correlation of size between donor and recipient is more important for heart-lung transplantation than for orthotopic cardiac transplantation. It is much better to have a donor with lungs that are slightly smaller rather than slightly larger, as smaller lungs will expand to fill the space whereas large lungs will be compressed and have the potential to tamponade the heart; more importantly they may collapse and become a reservoir for infection.

The donor operation

On arrival at the donating hospital, as for harvesting the heart alone, a further assessment of the donor's state is made before harvesting. If this is satisfactory then the heart-lung block is removed in coordination with any groups harvesting other organs. The heart, lungs, and trachea are fully mobilised, the heart is arrested with cold cardioplegic solution, the lungs are preserved with a flush of 500 µg prostacyclin E_1 followed by ice cold Euro-Collins solution, and the heart-lung block is removed by dividing the superior vena cava, the inferior vena cava, the aorta, and the trachea. The heart-lung block is then placed in a series of plastic bags, each filled with a litre of ice cold Hartmann's solution and placed in ice slush in an insulated box for transfer.

The recipient operation

Implantation of the new heart-lung block takes place on full cardiopulmonary bypass. The superior vena cava and inferior vena cava are cannulated separately, and the ascending aorta is cannulated. The cavas are occluded by snuggers, and the aorta cross–clamped. The old heart-lung block is excised in parts. Firstly, the pleura is opened wide on both sides, and the pericardium is opened well behind the phrenic nerves and just in front of the pulmonary veins, leaving the phrenic nerves well protected in strips of pericardium. The left and right main bronchi are stapled and then divided, and the vascular attachments to the heart are divided and the lungs removed. The heart is then removed, either by dividing the superior vena cava and inferior vena cava if the heart is to be used in a domino transplant, or the right atrium if it is not, and by dividing the aorta. Implantation of the new heart-lung block requires anastomosis of either the superior vena cava and inferior vena cava or the right atrium itself; the aorta; and the trachea after trimming the donor and recipient tracheas to the appropriate position, which is usually two tracheal rings above the carina. The lungs have already been passed into the chest through the windows behind the phrenic nerves and the operation is then completed by securing haemostasis, which can be tedious, and closing the chest.

Pulmonary transplantation

The first isolated lung transplant in a human was by Hardy in 1963, and of the first 38 patients to receive lung transplants between then and 1977 only two lived longer than a month; one died at six months and the other at 10 months. Part of the subsequent improvement in survival with single lung transplant has come about because of the use of cyclosporin A, but there have also been technical improvements, both in the preservation of the donor organs and in the operation itself.

Indications

Single lung transplantation was initially indicated for the treatment of end-stage pulmonary fibrosis, but it is now also becoming established for patients with emphysema and also those with primary pulmonary hypertension. It is avoided in cystic fibrosis because of the continuing infection in the opposite lung, and these patients are better treated either with bilateral single lung transplants, as opposed to en-block double lung transplants, or (preferably) with heart and lung transplantation, with its single tracheal anastomosis. It was originally avoided in both emphysema and pulmonary hypertension, but continuing experience and improving results, often driven by the pressures on donor supply for heart-lung transplant programmes, has shown that it is feasible in both these groups of patients.

Patients selected for single lung transplantation should have diseases that are not amenable to lesser procedures, be under 60 years of age, and without other organ disease, evidence of malignancy, or overwhelming sepsis.

Currently about 50 single lung transplants are done each year in the United Kingdom and about 200 a year in the world. With the increasing demand for this procedure and the continuing shortage of appropriate donor organs, techniques of lobar transplantation have been developed. These techniques are of particular interest in children, not only because they allow larger cadaveric organs to be transplanted into children, but also because there is now the potential for living-related transplants. In theory it should also allow a single cadaveric lung to be split between two appropriately sized children.

Risks and benefits of single lung transplantation

Early mortality from single lung transplantation is about 5% within the first 30 days, but a further quarter will die within the first year. Most of these deaths are caused by rejection, multiple-organ failure, and infection. Anastomotic problems in the bronchus can also be troublesome. Overwhelming viral infection with cytomegalovirus is no longer a serious problem as most units now use ganciclovir for prophylaxis against cytomegalovirus infection during the early postoperative period.

The one year actuarial survival is about 70%, but it is too early to make accurate projections of five year actuarial survival. Symptomatic benefit in the survivors is usually dramatic in the short and medium term, but in the longer term the effects of obliterative bronchiolitis have still to be fully assessed.

The operation of single lung transplantation

Donor selection is similar to that for other intrathoracic organ transplantation, being based on ABO compatibility, chest dimensions, and pulmonary function. Donor harvesting is as for heart-lung transplantation, and the heart-lung block is then separated into its component elements.

Single lung transplantation can be done without cardiopulmonary bypass, but it should be available for patients with primary pulmonary hypertension, pulmonary fibrosis, or emphysema. Before removing the diseased lung it is necessary to have a test period of one lung ventilation with the pulmonary artery cross–clamped. Cardiopulmonary bypass is required for single lung transplantation in patients with pulmonary hypertension. If repair of an intracardiac defect is required then the right lung is transplanted as this makes access easier. Otherwise either lung can be used, but usually the lung with the worse function on preoperative ventilation perfusion scans is replaced.

The recipient's own lung is excised by cross–clamping the pulmonary artery and dividing it just before its first bifurcation; clamping the left atrial wall adjacent to the two pulmonary veins; and transsecting them and joining their orifices to produce a single larger opening. The main bronchus is divided just before its bifurcation. Firstly the veins are anastomosed with a continuous 4.0 polypropylene (Prolene) suture, then the bronchus is anastomosed with 4.0 polypropylene. The posterior, membranous, part is anastomosed first with a running suture, and then the anterior part with interrupted sutures. The pulmonary artery is also anastomosed with continuous 4.0 polypropylene. After air has been removed the lung is ventilated with 10 cmH$_2$O of positive end expiratory pressure (PEEP) to prevent reperfusion pulmonary oedema.

Postoperative management of patients with transplants

The early postoperative management of these patients is in general similar to that of most other cardiac surgical patients. The major differences relate to pulmonary vascular resistance and fluid retention after transplantation. Crystalloids should be restricted, often to 1 ml/kg/hour for the first five days, with the aim of keeping the lowest possible pulmonary artery capillary wedge pressure to achieve satisfactory tissue perfusion. Frusemide 40 mg is given eight hourly intravenously for the first 48–72 hours. Dopamine 2–5 μg/kg/minute is given for the first 24 hours or until renal function is adequate and the serum potassium concentration is maintained in the range of 3.5–4.5 mmol/l. Isoprenaline 5–10 μg/minute is used both to maintain a heart rate of around 100 bpm, and also to reduce pulmonary vascular resistance. Most patients will require insulin infusion, both to counteract the high circulating concentrations of catecholamines, and also to counteract the effects of the immunosuppressive doses of steroids.

Immunosuppression for transplantation

Immunosuppression regimens vary from unit to unit, but most follow the general principle of triple treatment for a period, and then double treatment with pulses of steroids and other agents during episodes of rejection. The same, or similar, regimens are used for heart, heart-lung, and isolated lung transplantation.

A standard regimen is azathioprine 2 mg/kg at induction, methylprednisolone 1 g when the cross–clamp is released, followed by azathioprine 2 mg/kg/day daily which should be discontinued if the white cell count falls below 40 × 10^9/l. Methylprednisolone 250 mg eight hourly for 48 hours is followed by prednisolone 1mg/kg which should either be reduced over six weeks to a

Regimen for immunosuppression

Steroids:
- Day 0   Methylprednisolone 1 g at release of cross–clamp, then 125 mg intravenously eight hourly
- Day 1   Methylprednisolone 125 mg intravenously eight hourly
- Day 2   Prednisolone 1 mg/kg orally, decreasing by 5 mg/day

Azathioprine:
- Day 0   2 mg/kg intravenously at induction of anaesthesia
- Postoperatively   2 mg/kg/day as a single dose increasing by 0.5 mg/kg/day to a maximum of 3 mg/kg/day, and decreasing dose by half if white cell count falls by more than half or to less than $30 \times 10^9/l$

Cyclosporin A:

- Started when haemodynamics are stable with no evidence of renal or hepatic impairment. Starting dose 4 mg/kg/day orally in two divided doses, subsequent doses depend on whole blood concentrations.

- Weeks 1 to 6   300-350 µg/l
- Week 6 to 3 months   200-250 µg/l
- 6 months to 1 year   150-200 µg/l
- After 1 year   80-120 µg/l

- Patients with lung transplants receive cyclosporin from the first day, intravenously, with target concentrations for the first month of 500 µg/l.
- The intravenous dose of cyclosporin is one third the oral dose and it is given by continuous infusion.

maintenance dose of 5–10 mg/day or, as is more common nowadays, withdrawn completely. Depending on renal function, cyclosporin A is started after 24–48 hours in a dose of 2–4 mg/kg 12 hourly, and then gradually increased to target whole blood concentrations of 150–250 ng/ml by the seventh postoperative day; target concentrations are reduced after three months to 100–150 ng/ml.

Antithymocyte globulin may be used during the first 2 to 7 days, its dose being 2 mg/kg (for rabbit antithymocyte globulin). It may also be used if the response to the pulsed steroid treatment is unsatisfactory. Newer agents such as tacrolimus (FK506) and muromonab – CD3 (OKT3) are also exciting a lot of interest since they were introduced in hepatic transplantation. OKT3 is not useful as an induction agent, but is used for resistant severe cardiac rejection.

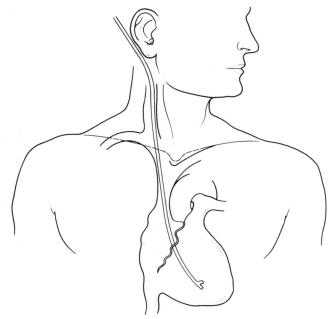

Figure 8.3 The endomyocardium is biopsied by inserting a bioptome through the right internal jugular vein and sampling myocardium from the right ventricle.

Endomyocardial biopsy specimens are taken transvenously for routine surveillance of cardiac rejection weekly for the first six weeks, two weekly from six weeks to three months, six weekly from three months to one year, and annually thereafter. If rejection is suspected at any other time then endomyocardial biopsy specimens should be taken urgently (fig 8.3). General malaise, low grade fever, signs of heart failure, and arrhythmias should all be considered as potential signs of rejection. The commonest problem is to differentiate between infection and rejection, and full bacterial and viral screens should be done if a patient with a transplant is readmitted.

Patients with pulmonary transplants have a different biopsy regimen, with transbronchial biopsy being less common. Home peak flow meters are used in most units for surveillance of early signs of rejection, and as for cardiac transplants, general malaise, low grade fever, signs of reduced lung function, and respiratory symptoms should all be considered as potential signs of rejection.

The management of acute episodes of rejection depends on the histological grade of the rejection. The principles are to maintain cyclosporin and azathioprine at optimum levels, and steroids are usually given as well as methylprednisolone 1 g intravenously once a day for three days. If necessary a short reducing course of oral steroids can be added. Alternatively prednisolone 1 mg/kg orally and reducing by 5 mg a day can be given.

Viral and parasitic diseases after transplantation

The common problems are cytomegalovirus and toxoplasmosis. Cytomegalovirus mismatch occurs when a recipient who is seronegative receives a heart from a donor who was seropositive and in such circumstances prophylaxis is given with anticytomegalovirus immunoglobulin 100 mg/kg intravenously, six doses at intervals of three weeks. Confirmed cytomegalovirus infection is treated with ganciclovir up to 5 mg/kg/12 hours, infused at a constant rate over one hour.

The main problems in lung transplants are viral and fungal infections, atypical mycobacteria and, particularly in the patients with cystic fibrosis, Pseudomonas infections. Toxoplasmosis is uncommon as patients with toxoplasmosis mismatch receive prophylaxis with pyrimethamine 25 mg/day for six weeks, together with folinic acid 15 mg twice weekly for six weeks.

9 Other cardiac lesions

- The aorta
- Cardiac tumours
- Pulmonary emboli
- Atrial arrhythmias
- Chronic constrictive pericarditis

Surgery of the aorta

Surgery of the aorta falls into two major groups, elective and emergency procedures. The emergency procedures are mainly for injuries such as aortic transsection, or for aortic dissection, and both are described in chapter 10.

Most elective aortic surgery in adults is either for aneurysmal disease or adult presentation or recurrent presentation of aortic coarctation.

Surgery of the ascending aorta

Aneurysmal disease of the ascending aorta, aortic arch, or descending aorta is, like aortic dissection, more common in patients with connective tissue disease or hypertension. Aneurysms of the aortic arch and aneurysms of the descending aorta are rarely operated on. Operations on the ascending aorta are a little more common, and are technically simpler than those on the aortic arch. They are also without the potential spinal cord complications of descending aortic surgery.

The general figure for replacement of the ascending aorta is a transverse aortic diameter of more than 5 cm, and the decision about whether to replace the ascending aorta alone or with the aortic root is governed by the anatomy of the coronary arteries. If the coronary orifices have "migrated" so that they are further above the cusps of the aortic valve than usual, and particularly if there is associated aortic regurgitation, replacement of the root is indicated. If simple replacement of the ascending aorta is undertaken there is a risk of recurrent aneurysmal dilatation of the remaining aortic wall in the aortic sinuses (fig 9.1).

The aim of operation is to replace the abnormal area of the aorta with a tube graft, and the operative strategy is governed by the anatomy of the distal ascending aorta. If there is a reasonable length of aorta of normal diameter below the innominate artery to allow positioning of a cross–clamp with normal aorta below the clamp, then circulatory arrest is not necessary. If there is doubt, a short period of circulatory arrest is necessary so that the anastomosis between the end of the interposition graft and the aorta below the aortic arch can be completed.

Operation for replacement of the aortic root

The patient is heparinised and a femoral artery cannulated. The chest is opened, the right atrium cannulated, and bypass instituted. The patient is cooled down towards 15°C, the heart being vented if there is severe aortic regurgitation. Between 28 and 30°C the aorta is cross-clamped and the ascending aorta opened, and cardioplegia is given directly into the coronary ostia. The anatomy of the aortic root is assessed and if the valve cannot be preserved it is excised and the coronary ostia mobilised on "buttons" of aortic wall. A suitable sized collagen–impregnated Dacron tube graft is selected and a prosthetic valve inserted into the tube if one has not already been fitted. The valved conduit is then sewn to the aortic annulus, appropriately sited holes are cut in the conduit, and the coronary "buttons" anastomosed to the conduit. Assuming that circulatory arrest is needed, once the patient's temperature reaches 15°C the bypass pump is switched off and the blood volume drained into the reservoir. During the period of circulatory arrest the cross–clamp is removed and the part of the aorta which was clamped is excised. The distal end of the Dacron tube graft is then anastomosed to the distal ascending aorta just proximal to the innominate artery. After air has been removed the heart is reperfused and the patient rewarmed.

The main problems during the postoperative period are bleeding, cardiac and renal failure, and stroke. The problem of bleeding has been reduced in recent years by the use of collagen impregnated grafts, aprotinin, and tissue glues such as gelatin-resorcinol-formaldehyde (GRF) glue. Cerebral damage is a potential problem, but as duration of circulatory arrest shortens with increasing experience, and techniques of cerebral protection improve, progress is also being made in reducing its incidence. The 30 day survival for an elective operation is more than 90%.

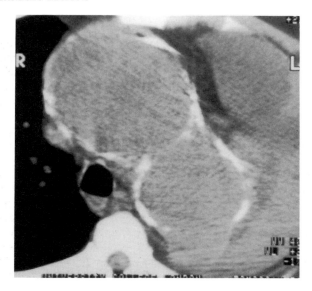

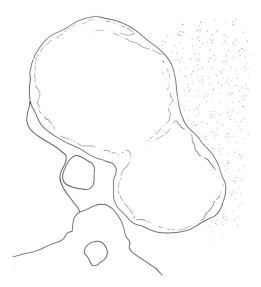

Figure 9.1 Aneurysmal dilatation of the ascending aorta.

132

Surgery of the descending aorta

Elective operations on the descending aorta in adults are usually for late presentation of coarctation of the aorta, for recurrent coarctation after repair in infancy or childhood, or for aneurysmal disease. The main problems are the risk to the spinal cord and methods to preserve its function rather than any particular operation. The arterial supply to the spinal cord is tenuous and its collateral blood supply unpredictable (see fig 9.2).

There are a number of different ways of managing this problem ranging from monitoring evoked potentials together with local cooling of the cord by placing ice along the back while the patient is on full bypass, core cooling, and circulatory arrest during the operation at one extreme, to simply clamping the aorta and doing the operation as expeditiously as possible on the other. Intermediate options include arch to descending aorta or femoral artery shunts (the heparin–coated Gott shunt is one example), and partial bypass, such as from the left atrium to the femoral artery. Each method has its supporters and detractors. Probably the most important manoeuvre is to ensure that the patient and relatives are fully aware of the risk during the preoperative preparation and that this has been fully and completely documented.

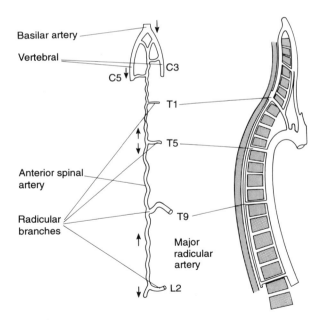

Figure 9.2 Blood supply of the spinal cord.

Cardiac tumours

Primary cardiac tumours are rare, and of those that do develop 70% are benign and 30% malignant. The commonest type of benign tumour and the commonest overall, is the atrial myxoma. This comprises 30% of all cardiac tumours. Benign lipomas, papillary fibroelastomas, and rhabdomyomas, and malignant angiosarcomas each account for 8–10% of tumours.

Atrial myxomas

Atrial myxomas usually arise from the atrial septum in the region of the limbus of the fossa ovalis, and 85–90% are on the left atrial side of the septum, though they may arise in other sites such as the atrial appendage or even the ventricles. They are polypoid or pedunculated, and contain a gelatinous core covered by endothelium. The cells are small and polygonal lying within a myxoid stroma containing reticulocytes, elastin fibres, smooth muscle cells, and collagen deposits. Atrial myxomas present in several ways, sometimes with signs of mitral stenosis caused by the tumour obstructing the orifice of the mitral valve. This may show itself gradually as worsening dyspnoea, or acutely as syncope from near complete or complete acute obstruction of the valve. Less often they present with signs of mitral regurgitation caused by damage to the mitral valve leaflets. Systemic embolisation of part or all of the tumour as the presenting symptom is common. As with the emboli that arise in mitral stenosis and atrial fibrillation these emboli can appear in any part of the circulation, as would be expected of an embolus arising within the heart. Occasionally the tumours present with systemic symptoms including fever, weight loss, and myalgia. Diagnosis is occasionally confirmed by histological examination of the tumour removed at peripheral embolectomy, but the most appropriate diagnostic tool is a cross–sectional echocardiogram, and the best views are obtained by trans-oesophageal echocardiography (see fig 9.3).

Urgent operation is indicated once the diagnosis has been established to avoid further systemic embolisation and mitral valve obstruction. About 50 operations for the removal of atrial myxomas are done each year in the United Kingdom, with an operative mortality of about 4%. The long term outlook

---

Presentation of atrial myxoma:

- As mitral stenosis
- Dyspnoea or acute syncope
- Systemic embolisation
- Fever, weight loss, and malaise

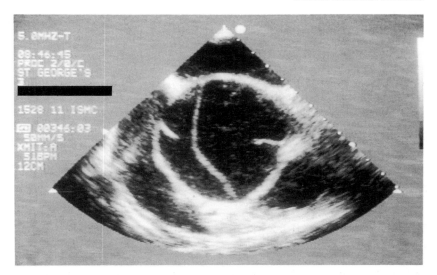

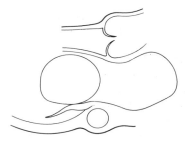

Figure 9.3 Left atrial myxoma seen on echocardiography. In this frame the myxoma is in the orifice of the mitral valve.

for survivors is good, though there is occasional local recurrence. Although myxomas are classed as benign tumours, distant metastases can occasionally occur.

Operation for atrial myxoma

Incision, cannulation, and management of bypass are the same as for mitral valve surgery, with the left atrium being opened through a standard left atriotomy. The tumour is identified and then the right atrium is opened separately. With the position of the tumour as seen from the left atrium as a guide, the septum is opened from the right and the tumour excised with a

135

Presentation of pulmonary emboli:

- Acute cardiovascular collapse
- Raised central venous pressure
- Classic $S_1Q_3T_3$ pattern on ECG
- Oligaemic lung fields on chest radiograph
- Pulmonary angiography is diagnostic but risky

---

margin of normal atrial septum. The septum is then repaired, either by direct suture or with a patch, and both atrial incisions closed. Air is removed from the heart and the patient weaned from bypass.

Other cardiac tumours are rarely operated on and management is tailored to the individual patient. Occasionally one may operate as part of a combined procedure with nephrectomy to remove the extension of a renal tumour from the inferior vena cava.

Pulmonary emboli

Pulmonary embolectomy for the treatment of pulmonary emboli has largely been superseded by thrombolysis with streptokinase, but may be undertaken acutely in patients with acute massive pulmonary emboli who are either too ill to survive while streptokinase is infused or in whom streptokinase is absolutely contraindicated. Usually, however, patients either die immediately from their pulmonary emboli or they can be supported adequately with volume loading and inotropes until thrombolysis is effective. Only about 20 pulmonary embolectomies are undertaken each year in the United Kingdom, and the 30% mortality reflects the desperate condition of these patients.

Emboli usually present with acute cardiovascular collapse, in association with high central venous pressures, often in a patient who is convalescing from another illness. ECG shows the classical S_1 Q_3 T_3 pattern, reflecting right heart strain, and the chest radiograph shows oligaemic lung fields. Pulmonary angiography though diagnostic is risky, as it may induce further pulmonary vasospasm.

The operation of pulmonary embolectomy

Either the pulmonary trunk can be opened using short periods of inflow occlusion, or cardiopulmonary bypass can be instituted; this is the preferred option. In either case the chest is opened through a median sternotomy.

If inflow occlusion is used, stay stitches are placed in the pulmonary trunk and both vena cavas are clamped. The pulmonary trunk is opened between the stay stitches and clot removed with Desjardins' forceps and the rough sucker. The stay stitches are then approximated to close the pulmonary trunk temporarily, and the caval clamps are released to allow the heart to reperfuse. The process is then repeated as required.

If cardiopulmonary bypass is available then the patient is cannulated and bypass instituted, though usually at normothermia and with the heart beating. The pulmonary trunk is opened and clot removed as above. In addition, the pleuras are opened and the lungs massaged in turn to try and move the clot retrogradely out of the segmental pulmonary arteries and back into the main trunk where it can be aspirated with the sucker.

Surgery for atrial arrhythmias

In the past there was a considerable practice of surgery for atrial arrhythmias, in particular the various forms of the Wolff-Parkinson-White syndrome, but the enormous advances that have been made in transvenous endocardial ablation of these accessory pathways means that now they are rarely operated on.

Chronic constrictive pericarditis

Pericardectomy may be done for chronic constrictive pericarditis, in which the pericardium becomes thickened and fibrosed. The process can affect all three layers of the pericardial sac, the parietal pericardium, and the layers of visceral pericardium on the inner aspect of the parietal pericardium and the outer layer of the heart, the epicardium. This can develop into a thickened and calcified mass that is not only tightly adherent to the surface of the heart but also constricting the heart, and preventing it relaxing and filling during diastole. A serious associated problem is the myocardial atrophy that develops. Acute cardiac dilatation and failure is an unpleasantly common occurrence in the early postoperative period. Operation is indicated on symptomatic grounds, usually signs of right heart failure with peripheral oedema, hepatic enlargement, and ascites rather than dyspnoea from left heart failure. The chest radiograph may show pericardial calcification, though echocardiography and computed tomogram are more sensitive. Cardiac catheterisation shows that end-diastolic pressures in the right atrium, pulmonary artery, and left atrium are all raised and equal.

Pericardectomy

An anterior thoracotomy can be used, but the approach is usually through a median sternotomy as this makes it easier to use cardiopulmonary bypass if required. The aim of the operation is to dissect the thickened pericardium off

137

the myocardium over the whole of the ventricles and the atrioventricular grooves. In the interests of safety, islands of pericardium can be left in place — for instance, if there is extensive calcification over major coronary vessels. The main postoperative problems are ventricular dilatation and low cardiac output, and inotropic support or balloon pumping may be required. About 5% of patients will die in hospital, but survivors generally do well.

10 Emergencies in cardiac surgery

- Penetrating injuries of the heart
- Blunt injuries of the heart
- Injuries of the aorta
- Aortic dissection

Introduction

The definition of an emergency is flexible, and of the conditions discussed below some always require urgent operation, some often do, and some can usually be managed medically unless they deteriorate.

Complications of ischaemic heart disease that are also considered as potential emergencies, such as operation for evolving acute infarction or complications of angioplasty, repair of post-infarction ventricular septal rupture, acute mitral regurgitation secondary to papillary muscle rupture, and rupture of the heart after myocardial infarction, are considered in chapter 6 as complications of ischaemic heart disease.

A common error in patients with injuries of the heart is to disbelieve the evidence of the injury. Cardiac injury is not universally and immediately fatal, and many patients with major cardiac injuries survive to reach an emergency department. Injury to the heart should be considered in patients with both penetrating and blunt injuries to the neck, chest and upper abdomen.

Penetrating injuries of the heart

The management of penetrating wounds of the heart has progressed since Boerhaave confidently stated in 1709 that "all wounds of the heart are mortal." Billroth wrote in 1883 that "the surgeon who should attempt to suture a wound of the heart would lose the respect of his colleagues." Aspiration of tamponade after a sword wound was first reported by Dupuytren in 1826 when he unsuccessfully attempted to save the life of the Duc de Berri, but it was not until 1829 that Larrey successfully "decompressed a wounded human heart by aspiration." The first successful suture of a cardiac wound was by Rehn in 1896, though Tourby in 1642 had reported finding a healed cardiac wound in a man who had been stabbed four years earlier.

Penetrating injuries to the heart are often associated with penetrating wounds of the precordium. The high risk area is bounded on the left side by a vertical line drawn over the left nipple, above by a horizontal line running over the sternomanubrial junction, on the right side by a line along the right border of the sternum, and below by a second horizontal line along the level of the xiphisternum. Injury to the heart must also be considered in patients with deep penetrating wounds of the rest of the chest, the neck, and the upper abdomen. Any part of the heart or great vessels can be injured, but the relative incidence of penetrating injuries of any particular cardiac chamber corresponds to the degree of exposure of that chamber to the anterior chest wall. The right ventricle is the most commonly injured chamber, followed by the left ventricle, the right atrium, left atrium, and then the great vessels. In civilian practice most of these injuries are caused by knives which usually

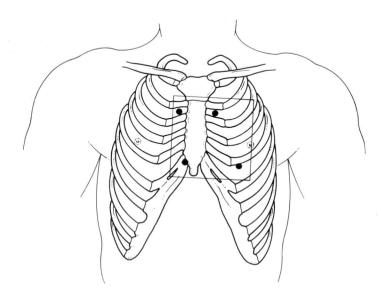

Figure 10.1 The "high risk" area for penetrating chest injuries.

affect only a single chamber. Bullet injuries usually affect more than one chamber, cause more damage, and have a higher mortality (see fig 10.1).

The clinical presentation of a penetrating cardiac wound depends on the severity of the injury and in particular on the state of the pericardial wound. A small wound to the heart may cause only limited bleeding, and if the pericardial wound seals spontaneously the patient will gradually develop the symptoms and signs of cardiac tamponade. If the pericardium is widely open (say, as far as the pleura) the patient will bleed into the pleura and the pericardial space will be decompressed. Instead of signs of cardiac tamponade the patient would instead develop signs of hypovolaemia. Larger wounds will cause more rapid development of signs and symptoms, but again if the pericardium is "closed", perhaps by clot over the wound in it, the signs of tamponade will develop rapidly. On the other hand, if the pericardium is open (either to the exterior or to the pleural space), the signs of hypovolaemia will predominate.

Tamponade is characterised by confusion, cool peripheries, hypotension, and tachycardia. The jugular venous pressure is considerably elevated, and the heart sounds may be muffled. The urine output is reduced, though treatment should have been initiated before serial measurements are made. Occasionally when the diagnosis is uncertain, echocardiography can be useful in establishing the presence of pericardial fluid. Pericardiocentesis may occasionally produce confirmatory evidence of cardiac tamponade and provide temporary haemodynamic benefit, particularly in those patients with minor wounds of the heart who are essentially well at the time of presentation and in whom the diagnosis of cardiac injury may seriously be questioned. Periocardiocentesis should be preceded by diagnostic echocardiography, however, and the increasing availability of echocardiography means that "blind" pericardiocentesis is hardly ever done. It is of little, if any, use in patients with massive amounts of blood clot around the heart, particularly if they have continuing bleeding from the heart. These patients require surgical

---

Cardiac trauma

Be willing to believe that the heart is damaged
ABC resuscitation (*a*irways, *b*reathing, *c*irculation)
Median sternotomy is the incision of choice
(Gigli saw passed on long Roberts forceps behind the sternum)
Consider intracardiac injuries, for late repair

Signs and symptoms of cardiac tamponade:

- Confusion
- Hypotension
- Tachycardia

- Cold peripheries
- Raised jugular venous pressure
- Reduced urine output

---

exploration without delay and pericardiocentesis may delay the definitive procedure.

The management of patients with suspected penetrating injuries must follow the classic "ABC of resuscitation", with attention to the airway, the breathing, and the circulation. These patients should be managed by a team, with an anaesthetist responsible for the airway and breathing, and another experienced doctor inserting preferably two large bore peripheral cannulas for rapid volume transfusion. If time allows, cannulas for monitoring central venous and arterial pressure can be inserted, but this step must not delay the appropriate surgical intervention.

In a patient with profound circulatory collapse and a penetrating wound in the high risk area, urgent exposure of the heart is required with internal massage if indicated, followed by cardiac repair. Determined resuscitation must be continued while the chest is being opened. If the penetrating wound is outside the high risk area but there is documented evidence, such as the weapon involved, which suggests that cardiac injury is likely, urgent exposure of the heart is appropriate. If the patient has a penetrating wound in the high risk area and presents with either relatively stable circulation or stable circulation after resuscitation then transfer to the operating theatre for urgent sternotomy is usually indicated. If the penetrating wound is outside the high risk area and the patient has stable circulation after resuscitation, a chest drain should be inserted for thoracic injuries and the rate of bleeding monitored. For abdominal injuries laparotomy is usually indicated.

A patient with profound circulatory collapse and a penetrating wound outside the high risk area and in whom cardiac injury is unlikely because of the site of the wound or documented evidence of the weapon involved, should have aggressive resuscitation and rapid reassessment. If the circulation shows signs of rapid improvement when a large bore chest drain is inserted, a further short period of reassessment may follow. If there is the least doubt, particularly in wounds of the left chest, then rapid thoracotomy is indicated to exclude damage to the great vessels.

A patient without profound circulatory collapse whose penetrating wound lies outside the high risk area and in whom cardiac injury is unlikely because of the site of the wound or documented evidence of the weapon involved, should have appropriate resuscitation and rapid reassessment. These patients can usually be managed initially with a large bore intercostal underwater seal

> ## Management of penetrating injuries
>
> - Circulatory collapse *plus* penetrating wound in high risk area:
>   Immediate operation
> - Circulatory collapse, wound *not* in high risk area, *but* cardiac injury likely:
>   Immediate operation
> - Circulatory collapse, wound not in high risk area, cardiac injury unlikely:
>   Resuscitation, reassessment, chest drain; if no improvement, thoracotomy
> - Wound in high risk area, but circulation stable:
>   Prepare theatre for sternotomy
> - Wound not in high risk area, and circulation stable:
>   Insert chest drain, monitor bleeding, and reassess

drain if they have a thoracic injury. The measurement of the drainage from the chest together with serial chest radiographs will indicate operative intervention.

Operating on penetrating injuries

The surgical approach depends on the site of the penetrating injuries and the surgeon's experience. For injuries in high risk areas most experienced surgeons use a median sternotomy. For injuries that seem to be lateral to the high risk area a thoracotomy is used. As most surgeons can do an anterolateral thoracotomy quickly this has been the generally recommended route for those less familiar with cardiothoracic operating. The advantages of the median sternotomy are that in the right setting it is quick and provides excellent exposure to the heart, ascending aorta, pulmonary trunk, vena cavas, and innominate (left brachiocephalic) and left common carotid arteries. The left anterolateral thoracotomy provides good exposure of the left side of the heart and can be extended posteriorly to expose the hilum of the lung, the left subclavian artery, and the descending aorta. The right side of the heart is best approached through a median sternotomy, as a right thoracotomy is usually reserved for presumed non-cardiac injuries in the right chest.

The absence of cardiopulmonary bypass equipment should not inhibit attempts at life-saving procedures; at the worst haemostasis should be attempted and resuscitation continued while efforts are made either to bring cardiopulmonary bypass equipment to the patient or to resuscitate the patient to the point where transfer is possible for a definitive repair.

Blunt injuries of the heart

The reported incidence of blunt injuries that cause contusion and other forms of cardiac damage varies, but is probably higher than generally appreciated. Cardiac contusion has been reported to be the injury most often responsible for accidental deaths and can arise from any form of blow to the chest. Cardiac contusions were rare before the advent of the motor car, and one of the first descriptions was by Schnabel who in 1859 described a 49 year old workman who died after severe blunt trauma to the chest. At autopsy he had "mediastinal haematoma, haemorrhages on the anterior wall of the right atrium, on the anterior wall of the left ventricle, and also an aortic tear". A necropsy study of unselected victims of road traffic accidents has shown the incidence of cardiac trauma to be between 15% and 17%, although if there are severe injuries to the body the incidence can reach 76%.

The usual mechanisms of damage are either violent contact between the heart and the posterior aspect of the sternum, or the crushing of the heart between the sternum and the vertebral column. In the first form of injury, the more rapidly the heart comes into contact with the back of the sternum (either by the sternum being driven backwards by a direct blow, or the heart being flung forward by rapid deceleration), then the more likely is injury to occur, and the more severe the injury will be. Similarly the rate at which the heart is squeezed between the sternum and the vertebral column, and the state of filling of the ventricles will affect the degree of cardiac damage in the second example.

The appearance of the heart will vary according to the amount of energy transferred to it during the injury. In a minor injury the damage will be limited to small petechial spots or minor bruising to the anterior wall of the left ventricle, whereas complete rupture of the heart can occur after a severe injury. Midway between these are coronary artery occlusion, and occlusion of saphenous vein coronary artery bypass grafts has been seen. Such patients present either with the changes of acute myocardial infarction or with angina soon after the injury. Minor contusions can be identified by non-specific ECG changes, which often resolve spontaneously. Patients with massive cardiac rupture die quickly at the time of their injury. Almost all patients who have appreciable myocardial injuries have some form of abnormality of cardiac rhythm, usually atrial or ventricular ectopics. In a patient with a heart that is not ruptured but who has evidence of myocardial contusion the usual cause of death is ventricular tachycardia or fibrillation. There is a small subset of patients with blunt cardiac trauma who have surgically remediable mechanical lesions, such as rupture of the interventricular septum or of the cardiac valves.

If a patient has symptoms from a myocardial contusion the most common presenting feature is angina–like pain that does not respond to vasodilator drugs. Some patients may complain of palpitations and show signs of acute myocardial infarction, including heart failure. Those with serious intra-cardiac mechanical lesions may present with the symptoms and signs of acute heart failure in addition to the signs of the mechanical lesion itself. Haemopericardium with signs of cardiac tamponade may develop early, and a pericarditic syndrome may develop later.

Clinical examination will show a tachycardia with or without signs of associated intracardiac injuries. The ECG often shows only non-specific ST segment and T wave abnormalities. Measurement of creative kinase MB activity and nuclear isotope scans are also neither sensitive nor specific, though a good quality echocardiographic examination of the heart may be helpful. Probably the safest diagnostic pathway is a combination of ECG, echocardiography, and measurement of the creative kinase MB isoform activity or troponin T concentration and to repeat these tests serially.

The management of a patient with a suspected blunt injury must follow the classic ABC of resuscitation, with attention to the airway, the breathing, and the circulation followed by continuous ECG monitoring to detect arrhythmias. The presence of heart failure means that intracardiac injuries should be excluded. If there is intracardiac injury it must be repaired surgically. Continuing heart failure, with or without intracardiac injuries, requires the appropriate use of inotropes and vasodilators, together with diuretics and even mechanical left ventricular assistance if required. The presence of myocardial injury should not prevent anaesthesia for the treatment of other serious injuries, but it will probably increase the operative risk and therefore the proposed procedures should be assessed in the light of this.

Injuries of the aorta

Traumatic rupture of the aorta is a deceleration injury, causing 10–15% of deaths from car accidents. The intima and the media rupture, and continuity is preserved by the adventitia. If the adventitia also ruptures it is almost always immediately fatal. Only the small group of patients in whom adventitial continuity is maintained will survive, as long as they do not have other associated fatal injuries and survive surgical repair.

The commonest site of aortic rupture, or transsection, is just distal to the ligamentum arteriosum in the descending thoracic aorta. Many patients have been reported in pathological series who have ruptures of the ascending aorta, often just proximal to the origin of the brachiocephalic artery, but these patients rarely figure in surgical series as they generally die of associated injuries, including cardiac injuries, before reaching hospital. Rupture of the descending thoracic aorta distal to the ligamentum arteriosum is rare, whereas rupture of the aortic arch proximal to the left subclavian artery is a recognised, though unusual, event. The rupture is almost always circumferential, and can involve just part of the circumference of the aorta, or the complete circumference with considerable separation of the intima.

As the burst pressure of a normal aorta is over 2000 mmHg, the mechanism of aortic rupture depends on a number of factors. Firstly, in a rapid deceleration the relatively unfixed heart and aortic arch will move relative to the descending aorta which is tethered to the thorax by the

Traumatic rupture of aorta

- Deceleration injury
- Suspect diagnosis from history and chest radiographs
- Definitive diagnosis usually made on aortography, though varies by unit
- Classic site is just distal to the left subclavian artery
- Intra-abdominal injuries usually take precedence
- Control blood pressure, avoid hypertension
- Steeply falling survival curve without operation

intercostal vessels and overlying pleura. Secondly, the heart will pivot around the relatively fixed left main bronchus and left pulmonary artery, increasing the shear stresses. In addition, the ascending aorta will lengthen acutely and then contract, which creates a water hammer effect and greatly accelerates the column of blood within it. It is the combination of these forces that results in aortic rupture.

About 20 thoracotomies a year are done in the United Kingdom for trauma to the aorta and great vessels, and of these about 45% will die. Some of the deaths will be the result of associated injuries, in particular to the head or the heart. These patients will have been operated on in the hope that the coexisting injuries could be successfully treated, particularly as many of the patients are young. Some of these deaths, however, will have been because it was not possible to repair the aortic injury, or as a result of the inevitable complications of operating on patients with multiple injuries. Probably the major determinants of operative risk are the condition of the patient on arrival in hospital, the degree of associated injuries, and the degree of containment of the aortic rupture. The natural history of the condition must be balanced against the high operative mortality after repair of aortic injuries and most series suggest that as few as 20% of patients with aortic rupture reach hospital alive, and of these initial survivors perhaps only about 20% will still be alive if they have not been treated by the end of the first week after injury. Long term survival without treatment is rare.

Despite the high operative risk, long term survival can be achieved only by operating on these patients, and successful operation gives excellent prospects of long term survival from the point of view of the aortic rupture, though there is a small risk of paraplegia as a result of ischaemia to the spinal cord during the period of aortic clamping.

Before transfer and operation, control of blood pressure is of great importance; the arterial blood pressure should be kept below 100 mmHg, even if there are other injuries. These patients must be transferred with full arterial monitoring in place both to aid resuscitation in the event of bleeding from the aorta, and to allow pressure surges to be controlled.

The operation of repair of traumatic aortic rupture

The main decision in the operative management of these patients is how to protect the spinal cord and distal organs during aortic cross–clamping. The choices are simply clamping the aorta and sewing; inserting a shunt between the aorta proximal to the clamps and the aorta or femoral artery distal to the clamps; or using some form of bypass support. Bypass support varies from partial bypass between the left atrium and either the descending aorta or femoral artery, to complete bypass between femoral vein and artery with circulatory arrest under profound hypothermia while the aorta is repaired.

With the patient anaesthetised and a double lumen tube placed, if possible, to allow the left lung to be collapsed during the procedure, the descending aorta is approached through a generous left lateral thoracotomy, entering the chest through the fourth intercostal space. Tapes for control are placed around the aortic arch between the left common carotid artery and the left subclavian artery (after identifying and preserving the left recurrent laryngeal nerve), around the left subclavian artery itself, and around the distal descending aorta. Clamps are then placed at these sites and the haematoma over the aortic rupture can then be entered in relative safety. It is sometimes feasible to repair the ends of the transsection by direct suture, but it is more usual to insert an appropriate length of interposition graft to bridge the gap between the two ends. We usually use a collagen–impregnated Dacron tube graft. The advantage of these over the older pre-clotted grafts makes their use essential if an interposition graft is required.

Aortic dissection

Aortic dissection is relatively unusual, but has serious complications and a high mortality. The underlying pathology is that the media of the aorta separates into two planes, the false and true lumens, and blood passes through both. This change is most common in patients with abnormal collagen, including those with Marfan's and Ehlers-Danlos syndromes, and in patients with uncontrolled hypertension. They may go through a transient stage of stability with the leakage of blood controlled to some extent by the adventitia and the pericardial covering of the ascending aorta, and the adventitia and pleural covering of the aortic arch and descending aorta. Without treatment, however, the leakage of blood usually (though not always) proceeds to frank rupture and death.

Aortic dissection has been classified by DeBakey and by Shumway. In many ways the Shumway classification is the easiest, and the simplest way to remember it is that any dissection arising in the descending aorta and extending distally is type B, and any dissection involving the ascending aorta or aortic arch is type A. The DeBakey classification describes a dissection arising in the descending aorta and extending distally as a type III — the

Classification of aortic dissection

- Shumway classification
  Type A — affects ascending aorta or aortic arch
  Type B — arises in descending aorta and extends distally

- DeBakey classification
  Type I   — affects ascending aorta, aortic arch, and distally
  Type II — confined to the ascending aorta
  Type III — arises in descending aorta and extends distally

same as a Shumway type B — but separates the dissections involving the ascending aorta or aortic arch. Dissections confined to the ascending aorta are DeBakey type II, and those involving the ascending aorta and extending into the arch or further distally are DeBakey type I (see fig 10.2).

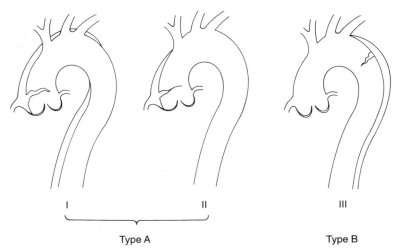

Figure 10.2 Aortic dissection. There are two components to the dissection, the intimal tear which typically runs about two thirds around the circumference, and the propagating rent in the aortic media, which is the dissection. There are two classifications. In the DeBakey classification Type I is a tear in the ascending aorta with a dissection running right round; Type II stops before the great vessels, and Type III is a tear beyond the left subclavian artery with a dissection running distally. A simpler classification, by Shumway, is to call all dissections which involve the ascending aorta — that is the most dangerous site — Type A and those that do not, Type B.

Presentation

Patients usually present with sudden onset of chest pain. The classic description is of a severe tearing pain that starts in the front of the chest and radiates through between the shoulders. Associated features are caused by major arteries being dissected off or obstructed, and these include confusion and neurological signs from impaired carotid flow, renal failure, and mesenteric ischaemia. Lower limb pain and ischaemic signs from dissection of the femoral artery are well recognised and can influence the sites of vascular access for aortography and cannulation for bypass. ECG changes indicate ischaemia, particularly from the inferior leads, after dissection of the right coronary artery, and they may also be caused by leakage of blood into the pericardial space. Prolapse of the aortic commissures as the aortic wall splits causes aortic regurgitation in Shumway type A dissections, and the aortic regurgitation can vary from trivial or absent to torrential.

Management of aortic dissection

The diagnosis of aortic dissection is initially made from the history and classic signs if present. The chest radiograph usually shows a widened mediastinum, often an enlarged heart, and there may be evidence of blood tracking along the mediastinal pleura on the left hand side. The confirmatory tests vary in sensitivity and specificity, and the choice usually depends on local availability. Transthoracic echocardiography can be diagnostic, but transoesophageal echocardiography is better (fig 10.3), though views of the origin of the innominate artery and part of the aortic arch are often impossible. Contrast enhanced computed tomograms of the chest can be useful (fig 10.4), and there has been considerable interest in magnetic resonance imaging but it is available in only a few places and the scans take longer. Digital vascular imaging is also used, though for many units the gold standard is contrast aortography.

Patients with suspected aortic dissection require continuous arterial pressure monitoring, together with control of their blood pressure throughout. This can best be done with intravenous infusions of esmolol and sodium nitroprusside, both of which are short acting and relatively easy to titrate against heart rate and arterial blood pressure.

Indications for surgery

The current view is that Shumway type B dissections should be managed conservatively with aggressive control of blood pressure unless the patient develops increasing pain or pleural effusions. A patient with chronic type B dissections who has continuing pain or a slowly enlarging aorta seen in serial chest x ray films, and particularly serial computed tomograms, should undergo elective operation.

Patients with type A dissections usually undergo immediate or urgent operations, the aims of which are to prevent further leakage of blood, particularly into the pericardial space; to stabilise the aortic valve, and to redirect blood flow into the true lumen by closure or excision of the site of the tear. For patients with Shumway type A dissections confined to the ascending aorta (DeBakey type II) this can generally be accomplished by replacement of the ascending aorta and resuspension of the aortic valve. If the tear is in the

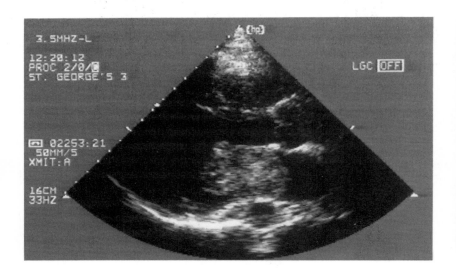

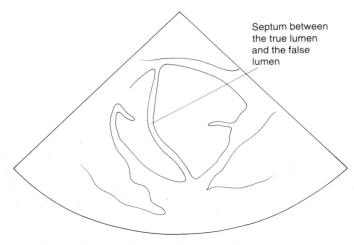

Septum between the true lumen and the false lumen

Figure 10.3 Echocardiogram of an ascending aortic dissection.

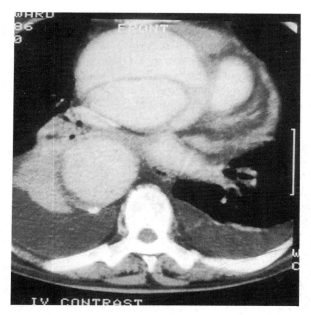

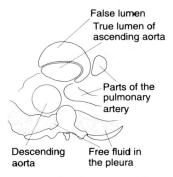

False lumen
True lumen of
ascending aorta

Parts of the
pulmonary
artery

Descending
aorta

Free fluid in
the pleura

Figure 10.4 Computed tomogram showing an ascending aortic dissection.

aortic arch, replacement of the ascending aorta will stabilise the aortic valve
and prevent intrapericardial rupture. If the tear in the aortic arch is identified
and this part of the aorta replaced, further leakage and distal dissection will
be prevented. If this is not possible then replacement of the ascending aorta
converts the dissection into a Shumway type B (DeBakey type III) dissection,
which can be managed medically.

Operation for ascending aortic dissection
   The patient is heparinised and the femoral artery with the better pulse is

151

exposed and cannulated. The chest is opened and the right atrium cannulated and bypass instituted. The patient is cooled down towards 15°C, the heart being vented if there is severe aortic regurgitation. Usually between 28 and 30°C the aorta is cross–clamped, the ascending aorta is opened, and cardioplegia is given directly into the coronary ostia. The anatomy of the aortic root is assessed and if appropriate the aorta is stabilised with gelatin-resorcinol-formaldehyde (GRF) glue, and the aortic valve is resuspended. An appropriate sized gelatin–impregnated Dacron graft is then selected and sewn with a continuous polypropylene (Prolene) stitch to the transsected aorta just above the aortic commissures.

Once the patient's temperature reaches 15°C the bypass pump is switched off and the blood volume drained into the reservoir. During this period of circulatory arrest the cross–clamp is removed and the part of the aorta that was clamped is excised, and the interior of the aortic arch inspected. If the tear has been excised at the lower end of the aorta, or if no tear is found in the aortic arch, the distal end of the Dacron tube graft is anastomosed to the distal ascending aorta just proximal to the innominate artery.

If there is an accessible tear in the aortic arch, that part of the aortic arch will be excised. This may be replaced with a separate piece of collagen–impregnated tube graft, and the tube graft is clamped proximally while the circulation is restarted and after air has been removed from the aortic arch. The two pieces of tube graft are then bevelled and joined together, and after air has been removed from the heart it is reperfused and the patient rewarmed. The duration of circulatory arrest is important and must be minimised (see chapter 2).

The main problems during the postoperative period are bleeding, cardiac and renal failure, and stroke. The problem of bleeding has been reduced in recent years by the use of collagen impregnated grafts, aprotinin, and tissue glues such as GRF glue. Cardiac failure, as after any other cardiac operation, is related to the effectiveness of myocardial protection and the existence of preoperative myocardial damage. Cerebral damage is a problem, but as duration of circulatory arrest shortens with increasing experience, and techniques of cerebral protection improve, progress is also being made in reducing its incidence.

The long term outlook for those who survive the operation is usually good, and reported survival rates in some series are about 80% at 30 days. The number of operations done in any one unit is, however, too low to make comparisons meaningful.

11 Congenital heart disease

- Classification of congenital heart disease
- Surgery for congenital heart disease
- Corrective procedures
- Ventricular septal defect
- Tetralogy of Fallot
- Pulmonary atresia
- Transposition of the great vessels
- Hypoplastic left heart syndrome
- Appendix: cardiac embryology

Classification of congenital heart disease

The most useful classification of congenital heart disease is that proposed by Anderson and Becker known as sequential segmental analysis. The components of the heart are described in turn, and then the atria, the ventricles, the great vessels, and the connections between them are described.

The morphology of the atrial appendages governs whether the atria themselves are right or left in type. The connections between the atria and the ventricles are then established. If the atria are connected to the morphological correct ventricles then they are "concordant", but if the atria are connected to the morphologically inappropriate ventricles they are "discordant". If the atrial appendages, and therefore the atria, are isomers their connection with the ventricles is described as a "biventricular and ambiguous" atrioventricular connection. If the atria connect only to a single ventricle then, depending on the anatomy, this is either a "double inlet" atrioventricular connection, or a "univentricular" connection. In the "double inlet" configuration both atrial chambers connect to a single ventricle,

153

Sequential segmental analysis

- Classify the morphology of the atrial appendages and describe the atria
  Left, right, indeterminate
- Establish the connections between the atria and the ventricles
  Concordant, discordant
- Classify the morphology of the atrioventricular valve(s)
- Classify the morphology of the ventricles
- Describe the morphology of the ventriculoarterial junction
  Concordant, discordant, double outlet, single outlet
- Describe the arterial valvar morphology
- Describe the morphology of the musculature at the outflow tracts
- Describe the relationship of the arterial trunks
- Describe the intracardiac malformations

whereas in the "univentricular" connection one of the atria is connected to a ventricle and the other has no connection with a ventricle.

The atrioventricular valve(s) can be identified by their relation to the ventricles and the relation of their tensioning apparatus to the septum. "Straddling" is present when the tension apparatus is attached to both sides of the septum, and "overriding" when the atrioventricular junction is connected to both ventricles. The degree of override governs the nature of the atrioventricular connection, the overriding valve being assigned to the ventricle that underlies its greater part.

The morphology of the ventricles themselves is governed by the pattern of their apical trabecular component, after which the morphology of the ventriculoarterial junction is described. Firstly the ventriculoarterial connections are established, there being four separate options. The connections between the ventricles and great vessels are normal or "concordant". The connections can be "discordant", with the left ventricle connecting to the pulmonary artery and the right ventricle to the aorta (as in transposition of the great vessels). There is a "double outlet" connection when both great arteries are connected to the same ventricle be it of right, left, or indeterminate morphology. The arterial valvar morphology is relatively simple and abnormalities usually relate to the number of cusps, their perforation, and their relation to the septum if there is a ventricular septal defect. Again an overriding valve is assigned to the ventricle which is connected to the greater part of the valve.

After this in the sequence the morphology of the musculature at the outflow tracts is described. The outflow tracts are both potentially complete muscular structures, but it is usually only the outflow tract of the right ventricle that is a complete muscular cone. The relation of the arterial trunks is described, viewing the aorta relative to the pulmonary valve from below. The position can therefore be described as anterior, posterior, side by side to the left, or side by side to the right. The intermediate positions are described as right and left, anterior and posterior. The position of the heart relative to the thorax is then described, together with the orientation of the apex of the heart. The sequential segmental analysis is completed by a description of the intracardiac malformations.

Surgery for congenital heart disease

The aim of surgery for congenital heart disease is either to correct the anatomical lesion (possibly as a staged procedure) or to palliate the child, either to allow time for it to grow before a corrective procedure is undertaken or as a definitive procedure in those patients in whom anatomical correction is not possible.

The aim of palliative procedures is to normalise the flow of blood to the lungs. Those patients who are receiving an excess of blood in the lungs, (those with a left–to–right shunt at atrial or ventricular level) are treated by pulmonary artery banding. Those patients who are not receiving enough blood to the lungs (those with pulmonary atresia or tetralogy of Fallot) have some form of shunt constructed to supply blood to the lungs.

Pulmonary artery banding

Pulmonary artery banding reduces the blood flow to the lungs. It is done through a small left anterolateral thoracotomy, entering the chest through the fourth or fifth interspace. The lung is retracted and the pericardium opened anterior to the phrenic nerve. By passing a tape through the plane between the aorta and pulmonary artery, and then pulling it back through the transverse sinus, it is possible to pass it around the pulmonary artery without attempting the dangerous manoeuvre of passing an instrument directly around the pulmonary artery. The band is then tightened, usually to a point at which the pressure in the pulmonary artery distal to the band is about a third to a half of that in the aorta. Pulmonary artery banding is effective at controlling heart failure, but less effective at reducing, or preventing an increase in, pulmonary vascular resistance. If the pulmonary artery band has to be removed later the pulmonary artery will have to be reconstructed.

Shunts

Shunting procedures are used to increase the blood flow to the lungs before corrective surgery, and probably the most common is the modified Blalock-Taussig operation. The original Blalock-Taussig operation is done

155

Palliative procedures

- Pulmonary artery banding
- Shunt operations
  Blalock-Taussig operations
  Modified Blalock-Taussig operations
  Glenn anastomosis
  Modified Glenn anastomosis
  Potts' anastomosis
  Waterston operation

through a thoracotomy on the side opposite the aortic arch. The subclavian artery is mobilised as distally as possible and divided distally. The divided artery is then turned down, the divided end of the subclavian artery is anastomosed end to side to the left pulmonary artery, and the origin of the axillary artery is closed. In the modified Blalock-Taussig shunt the subclavian artery is left intact, and a polytetrafluoroethylene (PTFE) graft, usually 4 mm in diameter, is placed between the subclavian artery and the pulmonary artery.

Other arterial shunts include that between the descending aorta and the left pulmonary artery (the Potts' anastomosis), and this is also done through a left thoracotomy. The Waterston operation (connection of the ascending aorta to the right pulmonary artery) is usually done through a right lateral thoracotomy (see fig 11.1).

The Glenn anastomosis is a connection between the superior vena cava and the right pulmonary artery, and the modified Glenn operation is a connection between the superior vena cava and both pulmonary arteries. This requires division of the azygos vein and (usually) ligation of the superior vena cava at its junction with the right atrium. There are a number of variations of these operations which can be selected according to the exact anatomical problem.

Corrective procedures

The principles of corrective procedures for a number of the commoner congenital defects are described here.

Patent ductus arteriosus

The chest is opened through a lateral thoracotomy through the fourth intercostal space. With the lung retracted forward to expose the thoracic aorta, the pleura is incised to expose the anatomy: the aortic arch, left subclavian artery, and the ductus itself, together with the vagus nerve and its

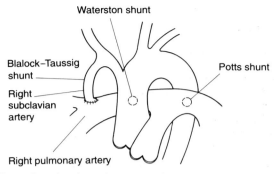

Figure 11.1 Examples of various shunt procedures.

recurrent laryngeal branch can all be identified. The ductus itself is closed by one of a number of techniques. It can be divided between clamps and the ends oversewn; it can be occluded by a clip; or it can be doubly ligated, usually without being divided (see fig 11.2).

Coarctation of the aorta

The chest is opened through a lateral thoracotomy through the fourth intercostal space. With the lung retracted forward to expose the thoracic aorta, the pleura is incised to expose the anatomy. The aortic arch, descending thoracic aorta, and left subclavian artery are identified, and the usual site of the coarctation is just distal to the ligamentum arteriosum. The

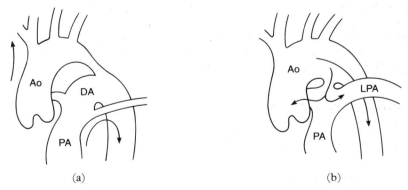

Figure 11.2 Persistent ductus arteriosus. In the fetus most of the systemic venous return passes through the ductus arteriosus (DA) to the descending aorta, and to the umbilical arteries to be oxygenated (a). At birth the ductus narrows and obliterates. If it fails to do so the shunt reverses and arterial blood passes into the more compliant vascular circulation (PA) (b).

157

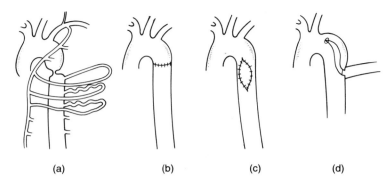

(a) (b) (c) (d)

Figure 11.3 Coarctation of the aorta. (a) There is a narrowing of the aorta beyond the left subclavian artery. An important part of the clinical picture is that the intercostal arteries from the third down, which arise distal to the coarctation, have reversed flow and shunt blood from the internal thoracic (mammary) artery and become dilated and tortuous, causing rib notching and a hum. Depending on the anatomical circumstances and the age of the patient the coarctation can be resected and the aorta repaired end to end (b), widened with a patch (c), or the subclavian artery can be divided, opened longitudinally, and used as an autologous patch (d).

coarctation can be repaired in several ways. The coarcted segment can be resected and the two ends of the aorta approximated and anastomosed, or the coarcted segment can be opened longitudinally, the obstructing membrane within it incised, and the incision closed with a patch to widen the aorta. Most commonly in children and neonates, however, the coarctation is repaired by the technique of subclavian flap angioplasty. The left subclavian artery is mobilised and divided, and the ductus arteriosus is divided and oversewn if patent. The coarcted segment is opened with an incision that continues up into the subclavian artery, following which the flap produced by opening up the subclavian artery is turned down and anastomosed over the incision in the coarctation segment to enlarge it (see fig 11.3).

Ostium secundum atrial septal defect

This is the most common atrial septal defect in which there is a defect in the fossa ovalis. To close it the heart is exposed through a median sternotomy, although a right thoracotomy can be used for cosmetic reasons. The ascending aorta, superior vena cava and inferior vena cava are cannulated. The cavas are snared, excluding the heart completely from the circulation, cardioplegia is given, and the right atrium is opened. The defect is identified and assessed, and can usually be closed by direct suture approximation of its edges. If it cannot be closed without tension by direct suture then it is closed with a patch, either of pericardium or Dacron. Air is evacuated from the left

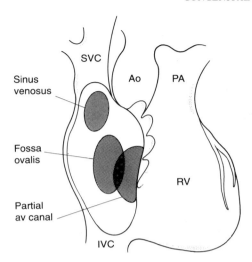

Figure 11.4 Sites of atrial septal defects.

atrium before the defect is finally closed. The right atrium is closed, the cross-clamp is released, and the heart reperfused. The patient is weaned from cardiopulmonary bypass and the chest closed (see fig 11.4).

Sinus venosus atrial septal defect

This is an unusual form of atrial septal defect which is usually associated with abnormalities of the venous drainage into the atria. The defect is closed with a patch sited so that the systemic and pulmonary veins drain to the appropriate sides of the atrial septum. The right atrium is closed either by direct suture or with a patch to enlarge the terminal superior vena cava. The cross-clamp is released, the heart reperfused, and the patient weaned from cardiopulmonary bypass.

Atrioventricular septal defects

In the normal heart the offsetting of the tricuspid and mitral valves is associated with a muscular septum between the left ventricular outflow tract and the right atrium. In atrioventricular septal defects the tricuspid and mitral valves lie in the same plane, with a defect in the position at which muscular septum between the left ventricular outflow tract and the right atrium should have been. The structure of what would be the atrial septum itself is relatively normal. The valve guarding the atrioventricular orifices is usually a common one containing five leaflets. The superior and inferior

159

bridging leaflets bridge the ventricular septum, with tensioning apparatus attaching to both ventricles. There are two leaflets confined to the right ventricle, the anterosuperior and mural leaflets. The remaining leaflet is confined to the left ventricle, and is also called a mural leaflet.

The ostium primum type of atrial septal defect is a particular variant of the atrioventricular canal defect that is confined to the atrial septum. Here the superior and inferior bridging leaflets are joined by a tongue of leaflet tissue, with the bridging leaflets attached to the ventricular septum. Because the valve separating the atrioventricular junctions still has five leaflets, the mitral valve was previously described as having a cleft anterior leaflet. In a complete atrioventricular canal defect the bridging leaflets do not attach to the crest of the ventricular septum and there is a common atrioventricular orifice. The degree of hypoplasia of the ventricular septum varies, but there is a bundle of conducting tissue running down the crest of the septum, under the cover of the inferior bridging leaflet. Further conducting tissue runs astride the midportion of the crest of the septum, usually covered by the connecting tongue of leaflet tissue.

Surgical management must be tailored to the anatomical lesion. The right atrium is opened and the defect identified and assessed. If there is appreciable regurgitation through the left atrioventricular valve, the valve is repaired by approximating the edges of the inferior and superior bridging leaflets. If the left atrioventricular valve cannot be made competent by this method, prosthetic replacement should be considered. The atrial septum is then repaired with a patch, using either pericardium or Dacron fabric. If the suture line is kept within valve tissue until it is beyond the orifice of the coronary sinus the conducting tissue should be avoided. Air is evacuated from the left atrium before the defect is finally closed. The right atrium is closed, the cross-clamp is released and the heart reperfused. The assessment of residual mitral regurgitation on the operating table is made by echocardiography.

The aim of operation for a complete atrioventricular canal defect is similar. The right atrium is opened, the defect is identified and assessed. The exact approach varies slightly depending on how much of the bridging leaflets are attached to the crest of the ventricular septum. If the left atrioventricular valve is regurgitant, the valve is repaired by approximating the edges of the inferior and superior bridging leaflets. If the left atrioventricular valve cannot be made competent in this way, prosthetic replacement should be considered at this stage. The defect is then patched, with the sutures on the ventricular septum being kept to the right side of the septum and below its crest to avoid the conducting tissue. Air is evacuated from the left atrium before the defect is finally closed. The right atrium is closed, the cross-clamp is released, and the heart reperfused. The assessment of residual mitral regurgitation on the operating table is conventionally made by palpation and study of the left atrial wave form, but echocardiography is being increasingly used.

Indications for closure of isolated ventricular septal defects

- Infants less than 3 months of age, severe heart failure:
  Early closure or pulmonary artery banding
- Children over 3 months of age with severe heart failure, and failure to thrive or increased pulmonary vascular resistance
- Children over 6 months of age with a persistent defect

Ventricular septal defect

The interventricular septum is a complex structure, with several parts. It can be divided into a small fibrous part, known as the membranous septum, and a larger muscular part. The muscular part can be subdivided into three portions known as the inlet septum, the trabecular septum, and the outlet septum. The trabecular septum comprises a larger portion of the interventricular septum than is at first realised, as it is a curved structure which forms part of the cone of the left ventricle. The right ventricle is a crescent shaped structure applied to the side of the left ventricle.

Because ventricular septal defects that present in neonates and infants can close spontaneously, not all defects diagnosed early require closure. For isolated ventricular septal defects, the indications for closure are generally as follows. If the infant is less than 3 months of age then closure is indicated if the child has severe heart failure. Occasionally pulmonary artery banding is indicated if the anatomy of the defect is particularly unsuitable for early closure (as in multiple defects). If severe symptoms of heart failure are present in a child over 3 months of age, if there is failure to thrive, or evidence of increasing pulmonary vascular resistance then closure should be undertaken at this stage. A persisting significant ventricular septal defect is unlikely to close spontaneously in a child of 6 months of age and closure should be considered to avoid the development of pulmonary vascular disease. The treatment of patients who present later depends on their pulmonary vascular resistance; increased pulmonary vascular resistance with evidence of reversed shunting is a contraindication to closure. Patients with moderately, but irreversibly, increased pulmonary vascular resistance and moderate shunting are difficult to manage.

Anatomically isolated ventricular septal defects occur in several different positions (fig 11.5), the most common (in about 80%) being the perimembranous defect. These defects are bounded in part by the area of fibrous continuity between the aortic, mitral, and tricuspid valves, which differentiates them from the ventricular component of an atrioventricular septal defect. The conduction tissue penetrates through the area of continuity of the aortic and tricuspid valves. Muscular ventricular septal defects may be

161

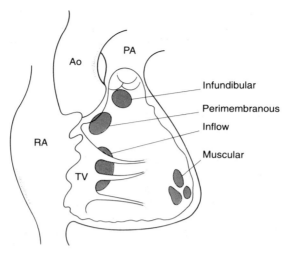

Figure 11.5 Sites of ventricular septal defects.

distinguished from the perimembranous defects by being entirely enclosed within the muscular part of the interventricular septum. The defects in the inlet part of the septum lie inferior to the conduction tissue, and the defects in the trabecular part of the septum can be single or multiple. A large trabecular defect can be crossed by the septomarginal trabeculum and seem to be a pair of defects. These trabecular defects are not related to important elements of the conducting system. Isolated defects of the outlet part of the muscular septum are uncommon In the doubly committed ventricular septal defect both the posterior aspect of the subpulmonary infundibulum and the muscular outlet septum are absent so that the aortic and pulmonary valves lie in continuity in the superior rim of the defect.

Operations for ventricular septal defects

Ventricular septal defects can often be approached by opening the right atrium and working through the tricuspid valve. Alternatively, depending on the position of the defect, the left or right ventricles or even the pulmonary trunk may be opened. In infants the use of deep hypothermia and circulatory arrest facilitates the procedure. After bypass has been started, the patient is cooled, the aorta cross–clamped, cardioplegia given into the heart, and the circulation arrested. The venous cannula is removed to improve access and the right atrium opened. By retracting the leaflets of the tricuspid valve carefully, the interior of the right ventricle can be inspected and the defect identified. A Dacron patch is trimmed to the appropriate size and inserted.

The exact suture technique and positioning of the sutures depends on the particular defect and its anatomical relationship to the conducting system. After the defect has been closed, air is removed from the heart, and bypass restarted to rewarm the patient.

Tetralogy of Fallot

Tetralogy of Fallot is a particular form of right ventricular outflow tract obstruction, the anatomical characteristic of which is anterosuperior deviation of the insertion of the outlet septum. This narrows the subpulmonary outflow tract and opens up a ventricular septal defect, resulting in a biventricular connection of the aortic valve. There is associated hypertrophy of the infundibulum of the right ventricle, which results in a constricting muscular ring, produced by hypertrophied trabeculas, together with hypertrophy of the septal insertion of the outlet septum. There is often associated valvar stenosis of the pulmonary valve, which should also be relieved at operation. The connection of the aorta varies from being mostly to the left ventricle to mostly to the right ventricle. The conduction tissue penetrates the remnant of the interventricular membranous septum, usually passing down the left ventricular side of the septum below its crest (see fig 11.6).

Operation for tetralogy of Fallot

If complete repair is possible without the need for a transannular patch, the operation may be done in infancy, with profound hypothermia and circula-

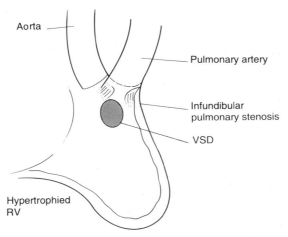

Figure 11.6 Tetralogy of Fallot (infundibular pulmonary stenosis, over–riding aorta, ventricular septal defect, and right ventricular hypertrophy).

163

tory arrest. Otherwise a palliative shunt may be constructed and the correction made in childhood when bicaval cannulation and snares will be used.

The heart is exposed through a median sternotomy and the anatomy inspected. The ascending aorta is cannulated, together with either bicaval cannulation and snares through the right atrium or (in infants) a single atrial cannula. Depending on the anatomy, the ventricular septal defect can be approached either through the right atrium or the right ventricle. If it is anticipated that a transannular patch will be required to widen the outflow of the right ventricle, a right ventricular incision should be used. After the obstructing muscle bundles in the outflow tract have been resected, the ventricular septal defect will be patched, taking care to avoid the conduction tissue.

The pulmonary valve will be dilated if appropriate, and the outflow tract of the right ventricle enlarged with a patch if its predicted diameter is too small for the size of the patient. Air is evacuated from the heart, and if it has been opened, the right atrium is closed. After further removal of air the cross-clamp is released and the heart reperfused. The patient is weaned from cardiopulmonary bypass, the heart decannulated, and the chest closed in the routine fashion.

Pulmonary atresia

The management of pulmonary atresia is constrained by the structure of the pulmonary arteries. Usually, though not always, the lungs are supplied either through a persistent ductus arteriosus or through aortapulmonary collateral arteries. Pulmonary arteries usually exist within the pericardial sac, and the aim of the preoperative studies is to define how much of the lung tissue is supplied by the intrapericardial arteries, and how much is supplied directly by collaterals. This governs the success of the attempted correction.

Pulmonary atresia exists, however, in two functional variants; pulmonary atresia with a ventricular septal defect, and pulmonary atresia with an intact ventricular septum. The more common pulmonary atresia with a ventricular septal defect is a variant of tetralogy of Fallot, and carries a relatively good prognosis, whereas pulmonary atresia with an intact ventricular septum has a poor prognosis. This is because the hypertrophy of the right ventricle that occurs in response to the severe outlet obstruction produces a range of cavities that are too small to function. The best prognosis is when the ventricular wall is less hypoplastic and the volume of the ventricular cavity is relatively well preserved. Usually in pulmonary atresia with an intact ventricular septum the pulmonary arteries themselves are of an adequate size and supplied by a ductus arteriosus which can be maintained with prostaglandin infusions.

Surgery for pulmonary atresia with ventricular septal defect

Surgery for this condition is similar to that for tetralogy of Fallot, and is guided by the size and shape of the distal pulmonary arteries. The right ventricle is opened and the defect closed. Then a valved homograft conduit is placed between the outflow tract of the right ventricle and the confluence of the pulmonary arteries, or (occasionally) the infundibulum of the right ventricle can be opened across the atretic pulmonary valve and main pulmonary trunk and a transannular patch placed.

Transposition of the great vessels

Transposition of the great vessels describes the heart in which the right atrium connects to the right ventricle, the left atrium connects to the left ventricle, the right ventricle connects to the aorta, and the left ventricle to the pulmonary trunk. In the terminology of sequential segmental analysis, this would be described as concordant atrioventricular connections, and discordant ventriculoarterial connections. Transposition of the great vessels is used to describe this particular abnormality, because other abnormalities such as double inlet ventricle or absence of an atrioventricular connection, can co-exist with, and dominate the clinical picture of, concordant atrioventricular connections and discordant ventriculoarterial connections (see fig 11.7).

There are two different surgical approaches to the management of these patients, either by an atrial switch procedure, or by an arterial switch procedure. The aim of the atrial switch procedure is to redirect blood flow at the atrial level by connecting the right atrium to the left ventricle and the left atrium to the right ventricle. The aim of the arterial switch procedure is to return blood flow from the right ventricle to the pulmonary trunk, and blood from the left ventricle to the aorta.

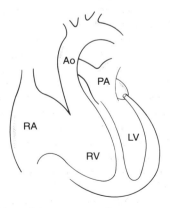

Figure 11.7 Transposition of the great vessels.

165

Operations for complete transposition of the great vessels

The arterial switch procedure is aimed at producing an essentially normal anatomical arrangement, by dividing the ascending aorta and pulmonary trunk. Cardiopulmonary bypass is instituted, the patient cooled, the aorta cross-clamped and the heart arrested with cardioplegia. Any associated ventricular septal defect is closed through the right atrium, across the tricuspid valve. The aorta is divided and the distal end passed behind the bifurcation of the pulmonary trunk (the Lecomte manoeuvre) and anastomosed to the proximal end of the pulmonary trunk (arising from the left ventricle). Next the coronary arteries are mobilised on buttons of aortic wall and transferred to holes cut in the proximal end of the pulmonary trunk, proximal to the suture line with the ascending aorta. The defects left in the aortic wall (where it arises from the right ventricle) are then patched with discs of pericardium before the pulmonary trunk is anastomosed to the proximal end of the ascending aorta (arising from the right ventricle). Air is removed from the heart as rewarming is completed, and the patient is weaned from bypass.

There are two different atrial switch procedures, the Mustard and the Senning operations. In the Mustard operation, cardiopulmonary bypass is instituted, the aorta cross-clamped and the heart arrested with cardioplegia. The right atrium is opened and the atrial septum or its remnant is excised, after which the coronary sinus is incised to direct its blood flow into the left atrium. A baffle is then placed so that the flow of blood from the superior vena cava and the inferior vena cava is routed away from the orifices of the pulmonary veins, across the atrial septal defect, and through the mitral valve into the left atrium. As this baffle completely encloses the orifices of both vena cavas and the atrial septal defect, the pulmonary venous drainage enters the right atrium and passes across the tricuspid valve into the right ventricle. The right atrium is closed and air is removed from the heart as rewarming is completed, and the patient is weaned from bypass.

In the Senning operation, cardiopulmonary bypass is instituted, the aorta cross-clamped, and the heart arrested with cardioplegia. Blood is baffled without the use of prosthetic material through a reconstruction of the atrial wall and the interatrial septum. Firstly, the free wall of the left atrium is opened to expose the pulmonary veins and mitral valve. Then the right atrium is opened with an incision that consists of three parts of a rectangle, the unincised base of the rectangle being directed towards the atrial appendage. A flap of the interatrial septum is created, also three parts of a rectangle, the unincised base of the rectangle being directed towards the free wall of the atrium — that is, the junction of the right and left atria. This atrial septal flap is sewn down around the orifices of the pulmonary veins, which directs the pulmonary venous blood towards the incision in the wall of the left atrium, and the vena caval return across the atrial septal defect towards the mitral valve. The lateral edge of the right atrial incision is sewn down on to the medial part of the atrial septum to complete the baffling of the vena caval flow into the mitral valve. Finally the rectangular right atrial flap is advanced to cover the incision in the left atrium, which directs the pulmonary venous flow into a new right atrial cavity and across the tricuspid valve into the right ventricle. Air is removed from the heart as rewarming is completed, and the patient is weaned from bypass.

Hypoplastic left heart syndrome

The hypoplastic left heart syndrome combines aortic and mitral atresia with hypoplasia of the left ventricle, ascending aorta, and aortic arch. In sequential segmental analysis it is described as an example of univentricular atrioventricular connections with a double inlet right ventricle. The aortic valve is absent, but the coronary arteries often arise from small sinuses of Valsava, and the hypoplastic ascending aorta provides the route for the coronary blood flow. The left ventricle is usually tiny and slit–like, and the inlet mitral valve is either atretic or extremely hypoplastic. Abnormalities of the aortic arch are usual and associated with a large ductus arteriosus which supplies the systemic blood flow. Coexisting coarctation is also common.

Surgical management is controversial: a two–stage repair has been described, but the long term results are poor. Transplantation seems to be the only alternative option, but although short term survival is promising, medium to long term results are awaited.

Appendix: cardiac embryology

The heart develops as a tube within the pericardial cavity between the 20th and 23rd days, and by this stage the tube has three layers — an endocardium, a myocardium, and an epicardium. The future atria are outside the pericardial cavity, and the tube within the pericardium will become the ventricles. As the intrapericardial tube grows much quicker than the pericardial cavity around it, the tube (the ends of which are relatively fixed) is forced to fold. At the same time a common atrium is formed from two paired structures and is then incorporated into the pericardial cavity.

As the tube folds, trabeculation occurs within two clearly defined areas, one part of which will form the left ventricle and the other part the right ventricle. Two venous channels (the left and right sinus horns) and their connecting part (the transverse portion) collectively form the sinus venosus, which in turn is connected to the common atrium. In time the left sinus horn remains only as the oblique vein of Marshall and together with the transverse portion as the coronary sinus. Meanwhile the right sinus horn is entirely incorporated into the atrium.

Septation of the atrium occurs as the atrium enlarges with a crest developing in the lumen of the atrium, the two limbs of the crest extending towards outgrowths forming at the junction of the atrium and ventricle. These are the endocardial cushions of the atrioventricular canal. The opening that remains between the primitive left and right atria is known as the septum primum, and this in turn is gradually closed by extensions from the superior and inferior endocardial cushions of the atrioventricular canal. Before closure is completed, however, perforations occur in the septum primum, and gradually coalesce, leaving the ostium secundum. As the right sinus horn is incorporated into the atrium, a septum — the septum secundum — forms to the right side of the septum primum with a concave free edge, and eventually the free edge of the septum secundum covers the ostium secundum, leaving a cleft between the free edge of the septum secundum and the septum primum, which is known as the foramen ovale. Uterine blood flows from the right side of the heart to the left side across the foramen ovale, but this flow is reversed at birth when the left atrial pressure becomes higher than the right. At this point the upper edge of the septum primum is pressed against the septum secundum, the two of which usually then fuse together.

Septation of the ventricles occurs as the ventricles dilate in the folded cardiac tube, pushing the medial walls of the two ventricles together. These fuse together forming the muscular portion of the ventricular septum. The great vessels develop from a region at the end of the heart tube known as the bulbus cordis. The proximal part of the bulbus cordis will form the trabeculated portion of the right ventricle. The mid-portion, known as the conus cordis, will form the outflow tracts of the two ventricles, and the distal part, known as the truncus arteriosus, will form the roots and proximal regions of the aorta and pulmonary artery. Septation of the conus occurs as swellings develop on the ventral and dorsal walls of the conus cordis and eventually fuse not only with each other, but also with a similar septum, the truncus septum, which has formed in the truncus arteriosus. This truncus septum separates the truncus into aortic and pulmonary channels.

As the truncus grows it rotates, and its distal part joins the truncoaortic sac, from which the six aortic arches originate. As it rotates and develops further the origin of the fourth aortic arch aligns with the aortic channel, whilst the origin of the sixth aortic arch aligns with the pulmonary channel. At the same time a thick septum forms between the origins of the fourth and sixth arches forming the aorticopulmonary septum, the edge of which meets and fuses with the distal edge of the truncus septum.

At this time there will still be a large interventricular foramen above the muscular interventricular septum and below the conus septum. This foramen is closed by outgrowth of tissue from the inferior endocardial cushions along the top of the interventricular septum. It later becomes thin and fibrous, and forms the membranous portion of the interventricular septum.

The atrioventricular valves form after fusion of the endocardial cushions has divided the atrioventricular canal into right and left orifices. Hollowing out of tissue located on the ventricular surface of the endocardial cushions leaves the valves which are attached to prominent trabeculae on the inner surfaces of the ventricles, which in turn become the papillary muscles. The ventriculoarterial or semilunar valves arise from swellings in the truncus which become hollowed out on their upper surfaces.

The superior vena cava develops from parts of two primitive veins, the right common cardinal vein and the proximal portion of the right anterior cardinal vein. The left brachiocephalic vein develops from an anastomosis that develops between the anterior cardinal veins. The suprahepatic inferior vena cava is derived from the right vitelline vein which initially drains blood from the liver to the heart.

The first part of the conducting system to develop is the atrioventricular node which arises in the dorsal part of the muscle around the atrioventricular canal, and probably the atrioventricular bundle (Bundle of His) arises from this before forming the right and left bundles distally. The sinus node develops later from an aggregation of cells at the junction of the superior vena cava and the right atrium, but the node itself does not appear until the right horn of the sinus venosus has been incorporated into the heart.

12 The postoperative period

- Postoperative problems in hospital
- Complications after discharge from hospital
- Quality of life after cardiac surgery
- Avoidance of reoperation

The postoperative period can be arbitrarily divided into in hospital and at home, and this depends partly on the particular postoperative day that is suitable for a given patient's discharge. Patients go overnight from the security of a staffed hospital ward, complete with regular observations of pulse and blood pressure, to a completely "unprotected" environment at home, and within the limitations of a medical system that is increasingly pressurised into "efficiency savings" this change of environment will tend to occur progressively earlier in a patient's postoperative recovery period.

Many patients are fit enough to be discharged earlier than they would have been in previous years because the technologies of bypass and intensive care have improved and they have less physiological disturbance. Before patients can be discharged home there must be adequate support at home; they should be physiologically stable, with a controlled heart rate and blood pressure; and have no fever or other complications. They should be adequately mobile, and for most this means that they should be able to go up a couple of flights of stairs with reasonable ease. Their wounds should be healing satisfactorily or should at least be healed enough to be cared for daily by a district nurse. There is clearly some overlap, but postoperative problems may generally be divided into those that develop in hospital, which tend to be medical, and those that develop at home which are split between "medical" and "social."

170

Postoperative problems in hospital

Particular early postoperative problems such as low cardiac output, low urine output, arrhythmias, and respiratory dysfunction are covered in chapter 4. The main problems that develop in the ward as patients mobilise are fluid retention, atrial arrhythmias, and wound infections.

Fluid retention

Invariably patients after cardiac surgery are overloaded with water, which is reflected by the weight that they gain postoperatively. Commonly patients will gain 2–3 kg, though some may have gained 5 kg or more compared with their preoperative weight when they are weighed 24 hours after operation. This usually shows itself as oedema of the non-operated ankle after coronary surgery, or of both ankles after other cardiac surgery. A leg from which a vein has been harvested always swells. In addition, the jugular venous pressure may be elevated and there may be sacral oedema. Some patients will develop both clinical and radiological signs of pulmonary venous congestion. In most patients this is easily managed with a low dose of a loop diuretic, such as frusemide 40 mg, by mouth for a few days. It is unusual for a patient who was not taking diuretics preoperatively to need them for more than a few days postoperatively. Graduated compression stockings and elevation of the legs are useful symptomatic measures.

Atrial arrhythmias

Atrial arrhythmias develop in up to 10% of patients after coronary artery surgery. They are usually reasonably well tolerated for a period, and generally respond to simple measures such as optimisation of blood gases, and giving potassium and magnesium as appropriate together with an appropriate antiarrhythmic agent such as amiodarone. This topic is discussed in detail in chapter 4.

Wounds and wound infections

Most wounds heal quickly and satisfactorily. Those patients who are at higher risk of wound complications include the elderly, those who are diabetic or who have been on steroids, the obese and those with chronic heart failure. Patients who have prolonged and stormy postoperative courses, particularly if long periods of ventilation were required, are also at higher risk of complications. The most serious wound complication is mediastinitis in association with a major sternal wound infection, but this is rare, the incidence being well under 1%. Erythema and serous discharge develop occasionally, but if the sternum is stable the patients can usually be managed

171

with antibiotics and close observation. A patient with similar signs and an unstable sternum should be considered for re-exploration and rewiring, particularly if they are feverish or have a raised white cell count.

Leg wounds made for the purpose of vein harvesting often cause more problems than the sternal wounds. The leg invariably swells and should always be treated with a compression stocking. Complications can be reduced if one avoids making an incision across the flexural crease at the knee and avoids continuing the thigh incision into the groin. Sternal wound complications are lessened if groin incisions are avoided, as there is evidence that organisms found in the groin can be transferred to the chest. It is not always possible to avoid groin incisions, however, particularly when there is difficulty in finding acceptable lengths of saphenous vein, or when bypass has to be instituted through the femoral vessels. Scabbing and serous discharge from the leg wound are common, particularly from the area around the ankle and the flexural crease at the knee. Our impression is that if this occurs after discharge from hospital many patients will be treated with antibiotics, although the risks of antibiotic treatment are greater than the benefits. The most appropriate management is dry dressings, elevation of the leg when sitting, sitting rather than standing, or walking rather than standing. Serious complications of leg wounds are comparatively rare, and tend to develop in patients who are taking steroids or who have pre-existing peripheral vascular disease, diabetes, or venous eczema.

The only problem peculiar to groin incision is an occasional prolonged lymphatic leak caused by damage to the lymphatic vessels at the time of arterial cannulation. It may require re-exploration.

Complications after discharge from hospital

It can sometimes be difficult to differentiate the occasional serious complication from the number of trivial events that can occur.

Wounds

By the time patients are discharged from hospital their sternal wounds are healing well and their sternums do not move when they cough. A discharge may develop from a sternal wound for a number of reasons. If the patient has a temperature together with a tender, mobile sternum then mediastinitis should be suspected and the patient immediately discussed with the surgical team. Such patients will need formal re-exploration of the sternal wound. This is a risky procedure and the patients must be fully informed and give consent. If the patient has no fever and only a localised area of discharge from the wound, it can be treated like any other wound infection by incision, drainage, and culture of any pus. Antibiotics should be given orally, and only if appropriate according to the sensitivity of the organism cultured. A recurrent localised discharge is often associated with infection around a sternal wire and indicates that the offending wire should be removed; this must be done by the surgical team.

Given the length of most wounds for vein harvesting (often the whole length of the leg), the occasional discharging point is not uncommon. Unless the patient is feverish or organisms have been cultured from the discharge, these points should generally be treated in the first instance with dry, absorbent dressings, compression stockings, and elevation of the leg, as discussed earlier in this chapter. Occasionally ties or pieces of stitch may be discharged through the wound, but this is now uncommon with the increasing use of absorbable stitches and ties.

Postoperative chest infections

Late postoperative chest infections (defined by productive sputum, fever, and clinical or radiological signs) are relatively rare. They should be treated with oral antibiotics, the choice of which should be confirmed by culture of the sputum. The antibiotic that we prefer is trimethoprim, but clearly choices will depend on the local flora. A small number of patients will develop late fluid retention that masquerades as a chest infection, but these patients usually have both bilateral chest signs and other signs of mild to moderate cardiac failure.

Patients who have had an internal mammary artery graft as part of their procedure may develop late pleural effusions on the side from which the artery was harvested, probably because the pleura was not completely drained of blood and clot at the end of the procedure and this gradually drew more fluid into the space. These patients usually have the classic signs of a pleural effusion and respond to pleural tap.

Chest wall pain

A number of patients complain of chest wall pain after harvesting of the internal thoracic artery, which is commoner on the left side than the right. It can generally be differentiated from postoperative recurrent angina because it is not related to exercise, it is exacerbated by changes in position, and there is often associated numbness of the skin of the chest wall, particularly in the parasternal region. Odd aches and pains are common, and they usually respond to simple analgesia and tend to be self–limiting. Severe pericarditic pain is unusual, and when associated with a temperature and raised white count as in the classic "postcardiotomy syndrome" it can be distressing, but it usually responds rapidly to anti-inflammatory agents.

Arrhythmias

Arrhythmias late after operation are uncommon, and the underlying cause should be sought. In particular, serum electrolyte concentrations should be checked. Occasionally there may be ECG changes suggestive of acute graft occlusion, or there may be clinical signs of a late cardiac tamponade. Echocardiography should be done to exclude pericardial effusion. Other occasional precipitating events include chest infections and pulmonary collapse. Treatment depends on the nature of the arrhythmia and the precipitating cause, if any.

Low cardiac output

Low cardiac output that develops in the late postoperative period is unusual. Investigation should exclude a primary myocardial event such as graft occlusion or tamponade in the first instance. Over–diuresis is another cause, but in such cases the jugular venous pressure will be low, in contrast to tamponade or a myocardial problem.

Confusional states

Confusional states in the early to middle postoperative period are unusual. The occasional patient who was unremarkable before operation will develop a non-specific confusion, occasionally with some belligerence. These are unlikely to last long and the usual investigations such as measurement of urea, and electrolyte concentrations and blood gas tensions, ECG and chest radiograph should be done, but are often unhelpful. The relatives should be asked about possible misuse of alcohol if this has not been previously established with the patient. Management includes reassurance, the appropriate treatment of any abnormal investigations, and then haloperidol or chlormethiazole should be given if indicated. Chronic alcohol misusers can often be managed smoothly during the postoperative period with a low dose infusion of intravenous alcohol.

The quality of life after cardiac surgery

Indices of quality of life can be difficult to define and have been extensively studied in recent years, mainly after coronary artery surgery but also after transplantation. Most of the younger patients should be fit to return to work after operation, and the older ones should gain more enjoyment from their activities during retirement. Any patient who was working before coronary artery surgery should expect to be fit to return to work afterwards. Some of those who were unable to work beforehand will be fit to work, though there is still a degree of uninformed prejudice that prevents some patients who wish to work from doing so.

Patients with sedentary occupations are usually ready to return to work by about six weeks, but those with more strenuous activities will take up to three months. If patients can return to work part time at first we think that they should, to give them time to regain confidence in their abilities and come to realise how few limitations they have. Motivated people, such as those who are self employed have a strong vested interest, and will sometimes return to work within four weeks, though this is unusual. If a previously fit patient needs more than three months before being fit to work then careful reassessment is necessary.

Physical activities such as walking should be actively encouraged from the time of discharge, and patients should return to normal patterns of sleep as soon as possible. Travelling by air is usually possible from about 10 days after the operation, but this depends more on the patient's general comfort than any arbitrary medical decision. To reduce the risk of venous stasis, patients (like any other airline passenger) should be encouraged to walk around during a flight. Perhaps this should be particularly emphasised in this group as they will have had periods of bed rest during the postoperative period. Sexual activity may be restarted when both the patient and partner are comfortable with the idea. We usually recommend that the patient should take a relaxed role in the proceedings, but our impression is that most patients sort out for themselves what they want to do and when.

The patient should not start driving again until after being seen by the surgeon in the follow up clinic at 4 – 6 weeks. Our rules are that patients should have informed their insurance companies that they have been successfully operated on, that they should be able to wear seatbelts in comfort, look back over their shoulders, and be able to do an emergency stop.

Recently the Driver and Vehicle Licensing Authority (DVLA) at Swansea issued a guide to the current medical standards of fitness to drive (*At a glance guide to the current medical standards of fitness to drive*, Medical Advisory Branch, DVLA, Swansea). Group 1 licences are the ordinary driving licences, and Group 2, the vocational licences that were previously known as HGV/PSV but are now known as LGV (large goods vehicle) and PCV (passenger carrying vehicle) licences. A summary is shown in the box.

(Re)licensing will normally be permitted three months after successful rehabilitation provided the person can SAFELY complete at least three stages of the protocol or its equivalent, while off all cardioactive treatment for 24 hours and remain free of symptoms and signs of cardiac dysfunction during the test. The licence will be refused or revoked if there is appreciable pathological shift of the ST segment during or after the test, or if the patient fails to achieve or maintain a rise in systolic blood pressure, or develops ventricular tachycardia or other malignant arrhythmias, or develops symptoms attributable to peripheral vascular disease that limit the investigation.

175

Cardiovascular disorder	Group 1 entitlement	Group 2 entitlement
Successful coronary bypass grafting	At least one month off driving after the operation. If satisfactory recovery, driving may restart. Licence until age 70 retained. DVLA need not be notified unless there are other disqualifying conditions.	Recommended not to resume driving until fully recovered, at least three months after the operation providing there are no other disqualifying conditions. (Re)licencing will be permitted if exercise testing confirms able to meet national recommended medical guidelines.
Valvar heart disease (Anticoagulant treatment does not constitute a bar to the holding of a licence)	DVLA need not be notified, driving may continue unless there are other disqualifying conditions. Licence until age 70 retained.	Recommended refusal or revocation if in the past five years there is a history of: (1) cerebral ischaemia (2) embolism (3) arrhythmia (4) persisting LV or RV hypertrophy or dilation. Otherwise licensing will be permitted subject to normal regular review.
Heart or heart-lung transplantation	DVLA need not be notified, driving may continue unless there are other disqualifying conditions. Licence until age 70 retained.	Recommended permanent refusal or revocation.
Congenital heart disease (mild or simple disorders). Complex disorders should apply to the DVLA for further information.	DVLA need not be notified, driving may continue unless there are other disqualifying conditions. Licence until age 70 retained.	Uncomplicated cases will be licensed. Complex cases are likely to disqualify but each case will be reviewed on its merits.
Marfan's syndrome and allied disorders	DVLA need not be notified, driving may continue unless there are other disqualifying conditions. Licence until age 70 retained.	Marfan's syndrome and allied disorders with aortic root dilation normally will disqualify. Apply to DVLA for full information.

For group 2 entitlement only: exercise testing = standard Bruce protocol or equivalent.

Coronary angiography is not required.

The above comments are taken from the DVLA guide. If there is doubt about a particular patient then reference should be made directly to the DVLA Medical Advisory Branch, Oldway Centre, Orchard Street, Swansea SA99 1TU. Further information for group 1 and 2 entitlements is given in the DVLA leaflets CLE 1133 and CLE 1111 respectively, which are also available from the above address.

Avoidance of reoperation

A question that is almost as common as When can I drive? is What can I do to avoid reoperation? The general advice is firstly to attend to the appropriate risk factors, and secondly to take aspirin. Patients should be screened before operation for hypertension together with diabetes, hypercholesterolaemia, and hyperlipidaemia. Any with abnormal results should undergo the relevant investigation and treatment. Obese patients should be offered the appropriate dietary advice. Patients should be encouraged to exercise during the postoperative period, and to continue this in their later life.

Aspirin

Aspirin is recommended for all patients who have had coronary artery surgery and who do not have strong contraindications to taking it. The currently recommended dose is 300 mg every day. Evidence of benefit from lower dosages is conflicting, and there seems little further benefit from higher doses. The use of dipyridamole for secondary prevention has largely been abandoned.

Index

accelerated graft atherosclerosis 115
activated clotting time 8–9
air emboli 14–15
air travel 175
airway management 34
alcohol misuse 174
alfentanyl 30
aminoglycosides 40
amiodarone 37, 171
analgesia, postoperative 30–1
Anderson 153
aneurysms
    aortic 130–3
    left ventricular 74–6
angina
    after angioplasty 67
    history 45
    recurrent 64
    surgery 53–4
angiograms
    coronary 46, 47–53
    left ventricular 4–5, 53
angioplasty
    balloon coronary 5
    failed 67–8
    laser 5
angioscopy 5
angiotensin converting enzyme
        inhibitors 111
annuloplasty 81
antegrade cold cardioplegia 20–1
antiasthma treatment 35
antibiotics
    chest infections 173
    endocarditis 98, 99
    prophylactic 101, 102
    wound infections 172–3
anticoagulation
    artifical heart valves 86, 101–3
    cardiopulmonary bypass 8–9
    heparin 8, 32, 33, 87
    warfarin 86–7, 101–3
antithymocyte globulin 127
aorta
    aneurysms 130–3

cannulation 9, 14
coarctation 133, 157–8
dissection 147–52
stenosis 88–9
surgery 130–3
traumatic rupture 145–7
aortic regurgitation 89–91
aortic root replacement 131
aortic valve
    anatomy 103–4
    repair 79–80
    replacement 89–91
aprotinin 34, 131
arrhythmias
    atrial 137, 171
    during cannulation 13
    postoperative 37–9, 62–3, 174
arterial blood pressure 26
arterial cannulation 11
    air emboli 14–15
arterial pumps 12–13
arterial switch procedure 165–6
arteriovenous shunts 41
ascending aorta 17
    aneurysms 130–2
aspartate 22
aspirin 31, 33, 64, 103, 177
asystole 28
atrial arrhythmias 137, 171
atrial fibrillation, postoperative 62
atrial myxomas 134–6
atrial pacing 38–9
atrial septal defect
    ostium primum 160
    ostium secundum 158–9
    sinus venosus 159
atrial septum 16
atrial switch procedure 165–6
atrioventricular canal defect 160
atrioventricular node 16, 18
atrioventricular septal defects 159–60
atrioventricular valve see tricuspid valve
autologous transfusion 32–3
azathioprine 126

bacteraemia 99
balloon coronary angioplasty 5
balloon mitral valvotomy 80
Barnard 112, 121
basal metabolic rate (BMR) 15, 22
base excess 28
Becker 153
beta-blockers 62
Billroth 140
Blalock-Taussig operation 155–6
bleeding, postoperative 14, 32–4
blood cardioplegia 20, 21–2
blood gases 28
blood glucose monitoring 31
blood transfusion 32–4
blunt cardiac injuries 143–5
body temperature
  postoperative monitoring 30
  reduction (cardioplegia) 15, 20–3
Boerhaave 139
bovine artery grafts 59
bradyarrhythmias 38–9
Bruce protocol 2, 3
bubble oxygenators 12
bundle of His 16, 17, 18
buprenorphine 30
bypass pumps 12–13

calcium channel blockers 62
cannulation 9–12
cardiac anatomy 15–18
cardiac asystole 28
cardiac catheterisation 4, 5
cardiac contusion 143–5
cardiac embryology 167–9
cardiac failure see heart failure
cardiac injury 139–45
cardiac output 27
  low perioperative 62
  low postoperative 39, 174
cardiac tamponade 26, 141–2
cardiac tumours 134–6
cardiac valves see heart valves
cardiogenic shock 76, 106–7
cardiomyoplasty 106, 119–21
cardioplegia (cardioplegic arrest;
  hypothermic arrest) 15, 20–3
cardiopulmonary bypass 7–13
  risks 13–15
cardiopulmonary failure 121
cardiopulmonary transplantation 121–4
Carrel 111

cell savers 32, 33
central nervous system damage 41–2
central venous pressure monitoring
  26–7
cerebral injury 15, 42
Chagas' disease (South American
  trypanosomiasis) 119
chest infections 173
chest wall pain 173
chlormethiazole 174
clinical examination 46
coarctation of aorta 133, 157–8
codydramol 31
cognitive deficit 15, 42
cold blood cardioplegic arrest 20
cold crystalloid cardioplegic arrest 20
commissurotomy 79
compression stockings 171, 172, 173
computerised tomography (CT) 5
confusional states, postoperative 174
constrained vortex pumps 12
continuous cerebral perfusion 15
continuous coronary perfusion 23
continuous positive airway pressure
  (CPAP) 28
  facial 34
Cooley 121
coronary angiogram 46, 47–53
coronary arteries 17–18
  anatomy 64–5
  angiograms 47–52
  risk factors 46, 57
  surgery 44–65
coronary artery bypass grafts
  grafts 56–9
  indications 53–5
  operation 56–9
  patient selection 44–53
  target figures 44–5
coronary artery surgery
  decision making 57
  emergency indications 66–7
  operation 59–61
  outlook 63–4
  perioperative death risk 61–2
  perioperative morbidity 62–3
coronary sinus 16
coronary stenoses, anatomical
  distribution 54–5
coronary stenting 5
cricothyroidotomy 35–6
cross-clamp fibrillation 23, 60–1

cryoprecipitate 33
cyclosporin A 112, 115, 124, 127
cystic fibrosis 124
cytomegalovirus 125, 129

data recording 43
DC cardioversion 37
DeBakey 147
Demikhov 111
dental procedures 102
diclofenac 31
digoxin 62
dihydrocodeine 31
diuretics 171
domino procedure 122
dopamine 29, 40
doxapram 35
drains 31–2
driving 175–7
Dupuytren 140

echocardiography 2–3, 93
Ehlers-Danlos syndrome 147
Eisenmenger's syndrome 122
electrocardiography (ECG) 1–2
    stress test 2, 53
electrolytes 28–9
emboli
    air 14–15
    pulmonary 136–7
embryology 167–9
endarterectomy 59–60
endocarditis 97–101
endomyocardial biopsy 128
endovascular ultrasonography 5
exercise test 2, 53
extubation 34

facial continuous positive airway
        pressure (facial CPAP) 34
femoral artery cannulation 11–12
fentanyl 30
fluid retention 171
folinic acid 129
Framingham study 110
fresh frozen plasma 33
frusemide 40, 171

ganciclovir 125, 129
gelatin-resorcinol-formaldehyde (GRF)
        glue 131, 152
gentamicin 40
Gibbon 8

Glenn anastomosis 156
Gott shunt 133
Guthrie 111

haemodiafiltration 40–1
haemofiltration 40–1
haemoglobin, preoperative 32
haemopump 110
haemorrhage, postoperative 14, 32–4
haloperidol 174
Hardy 111, 124
heart block
    pacing 38
    postoperative 62
heart failure
    acute 106–10
    chronic 110–21
    decision making 106
    incidence 110–11
heart-lung (cardiopulmonary)
        transplantation 121–4
heart rate, postoperative monitoring 26
heart transplantation 111–19
    blood glucose monitoring 31
    cardioplegia 20
    contraindications 113–14
    donor heart 115–17
    implantation 117–19
    indications 112–13
    risks/benefits 113–15
    xenotransplantation 111–12
heart valves
    anatomy 103–4
    artificial see prosthetic valves
    endocarditis 97–101
    repair 79–81
    surgery 87–97
heparin 8, 32, 33, 87
Hering-Breuer reflex 121
high dependency units 24–5, 42–3
homograft valves 84–5
homologous transfusion 33
hypoplastic left heart syndrome 167
hypothermic arrest (cardioplegia) 5,
    20–3
hypovolaemia 141

immunosuppression 126–9
incisions 6–7
inferior epigastric artery 59
inferior vena cava 16
    cannulation 10

insulin 31
intensive care units 24–5
interatrial septum 16, 17
intermittent ischaemic arrest (cross-clamp fibrillation) 23, 60–1
internal mammary (thoracic) artery 58–9
international normalised ratio (INR) 103
interventricular septum *see* ventricular septum
intra-aortic balloon pump 39, 106–9, 113
investigations 46–53
ischaemic arrest 20
ischaemic heart disease 66–77
chronic complications 74–7
isotope studies 5

Kantrowitz 112

Larrey 140
laser angioplasty 5
Lecomte manoeuvre 166
left atrial pressure monitoring 27
left ventricle 17
aneurysms 74–6
angiograms 4–5, 53
function 4–5
hypertrophy 88–9
impaired function 55
leg wounds 172–3
L-glutamate 22
lignocaine 37
Lillehei 121
long saphenous vein 56–8
Lower 111
lung failure
acute 121
decision making 106
lung transplantation 124–6

magnesium 62, 171
magnetic resonance imaging (MRI) 5
mannitol 15
Marfan's syndrome 147
median sternotomy 6–7
mediastinitis 171–2
membrane oxygenators 12
membranous septum 17
metabolic acidosis 39
metabolic variables 29

methylprednisolone 126, 128
microprocessors 43
minitracheostomy (cricothyroidotomy) 35–6
mitral regurgitation 94–5
papillary muscle rupture 72–3
mitral valve
anatomy 103
balloon valvotomy 80
repair 80–81
stenosis 91–3
surgery 80–1, 95, 102
modified Blalock-Taussig shunt 155–6
modified Bruce protocol 2, 3
monitoring, postoperative 25–32
morphine 30
multiple gated acquisition (MUGA) scans 5
muromonab-CD3 (OKT3) 127
Mustard operation 166
myocardial infarction
acute complications 69–74
evolving acute 66–8
mechanical complications 68–9
perioperative 62
myocardial ischaemia 55
myocardial perfusion scintigrams 53
myocardial rupture 69–74
myxomas 134–6

native valve endocarditis 97–8
nephrotoxic agents 40
neuropsychological effects 15, 42
New York Association Functional Classification 2
nimodipine 15

obesity 46
obliterative bronchiolitis 123
oedema 171
organ damage 42
ostium primum atrial septal defect 160
ostium secundum atrial septal defect 158–9
oxygenators 12

pacing, postoperative 38–9
palliative procedures 155–6
papavaretum 30
papillary muscle rupture 72–4
paracetamol 31
parasitic infections 129

patent ductus arteriosus 156–7
patient controlled analgesia 31
patient history 45–6
penetrating cardiac injuries 139–43
percutaneous balloon dilatation 5
perfusionists 13
pericardectomy 137–8
pericardiocentesis 141–2
pericarditis, chronic constrictive 137–8
pH 28
platelets
  depletion 14
  transfusion 33
pleural effusions 173
polytetrafluoroethylene (PTFE) grafts
  59, 156
positive end expiratory pressure (PEEP)
  28
postcardiotomy syndrome 173
postinfarction ventricular septal rupture
  defect 70–2, 106
postoperative period airway
  management 34
  analgesia 30–31
  arrhythmias 37–9, 62–3, 174
  haemorrhage 14, 32–4
  monitoring 25–32
  pacing 38–9
  problems 170–4
potassium 28–9, 171
  cardioplegia 20
Potts' anastomosis 156
prednisolone 126, 129
prognosis 54–5
prostaglandin antagonists 31
prosthetic valves 81–7
  see also heart valves
  anticoagulation 86, 101–3
  dysfunction/failure 100-1
  endocarditis 98–101
  homograft 84–5
  replacement 101
  Starr-Edwards 98, 100
  xenograft 83–4
protamine sulphate 8–9, 32, 33
Pseudomonas infections 129
pulmonary artery banding 155
pulmonary artery pressure monitoring
  27, 39
pulmonary arteries 17
pulmonary atresia 164–5
pulmonary emboli 136–7

pulmonary failure see lung failure
pulmonary transplantation 124–6
pulmonary valve 17
  anatomy 104
  disease 97
  repair 81
pulmonary veins 17
pyrimethamine 129

quality of life, postoperative 174–7

Rehn 140
Reitz 121
renal failure 40
renal function 29–30
renal support, postoperative 40–1
respiratory dysfunction 34–7
respiratory variables 29
resuscitation 142
retrograde cold cardioplegia 21
right gastroepiploic artery 59
risk factors 46, 57
roller pumps 12
rotablation 5

saphenous veins 46
Schnabel 144
Seldinger technique 107–8
Senning operation 166
sequential segmental analysis 153–5
sexual activity 175
Shumway 111, 112, 147
shunt operations 155–6
sinus bradycardia 38
sinus node 16, 18
sinus venosus atrial septal defect 159
smoking 46
South American trypanosomiasis 119
spinal cord, blood supply 133
Starr-Edwards valve 98, 100
steroids 15, 31
streptokinase 136
stress (exercise) ECG 2, 53
stroke 41–2
  history 46
subendocardial scars 76
suckers 13
superior vena cava 16
  cannulation 10
supraventricular crest 17
supraventricular tachycardia,
  postoperative 62

Swan-Ganz catheters 27
synthetic grafts 59

tachyarrhythmias 28, 37
tacrolimus (FK506) 127
tamponade 26, 141–2
tendon of Todaro 16, 18
tetralogy of Fallot 163–4
thallium scans 5
thiopentone 15
thromboembolism 86
thrombolysis 136
total circulatory arrest 15
Tourby 140
toxoplasmosis 129
tracheostomy 36–7, 42
tranexamic acid 33
transient ischaemic attacks 46
transoesophageal echocardiography 3,
    93
transplantation 105–6
  cardiopulmonary (heart-lung) 121–4
  endomyocardial biopsy 128
  heart see heart transplantation
  immunosuppression 126–9
  lung 124–6
  postoperative management 126–9
  rejection 126–9
  viral/parasitic diseases 129
transposition of great vessels 165–7
tricuspid (atrioventricular) valve 16
  anatomy 104
  regurgitation 96–7
  repair 81
  stenosis 96

surgery 96–7
trimethoprim 173
tumours 134–6

ultrasonography, endovascular 5
urinary catheters 29–30
urine output
  low postoperative 40
  monitoring 28–30

valves see heart valves
venovenous shunts 41
ventilation, postoperative 25
  prolonged 34
ventricular arrhythmias, postoperative
    62
ventricular assist devices 39, 109
ventricular fibrillation (VF) 37
ventricular pacing 38–9
ventricular septum 17
  defects 161–3
  rupture (postinfarction ventricular
      septal rupture defect) 70–2, 106
ventricular tachycardia (VT) 37, 76–7
vents 13
viral infections 129

warfarin 86–7, 101–3
warm blood reperfusion 22–3
Waterston operation 156
Wolff-Parkinson-White syndrome 137
wound drainage 31–2
wound infections 171–3

xenograft valves 83–4

Cardiology books from the BMJ Publishing Group

CARDIAC REHABILITATION
Edited by Dee Jones, Robert West
Cardiac rehabilitation is coming into its own after years of controversy over its usefulness for either chronic heart disease or recently operated patients. In this book a respected group of specialists from Britain, Europe, and Canada evaluates the effects of rehabilitation and gives practical advice on its implementation.
ISBN 0 7279 0852 9   264 pages   1995

CLINICAL ECHOCARDIOGRAPHY
John Chambers
Perhaps the first book to put this major diagnostic tool into its clinical context, *Clinical Echocardiography* begins with a brief introduction on the technology followed by chapters on all the different disease patterns. Each one discusses the indications and gives many examples of echocardiograms showing the diseases. This concise text atlas is at the time a cardiology text and an introduction to echocardiography, containing over 400 illustrations.
ISBN 0 7279 0810 3   272 pages   1995

For further details of these books and our full range of titles write to Marketing Department, BMJ Publishing Group, BMA House, Tavistock Square, London WC1H 9JR
or telephone Diana Chapple on 0171 383 6541